D1528860

Lithium

Actions and Mechanisms

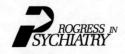

Number 50

David Spiegel, M.D.
Series Editor

Lithium

Actions and Mechanisms

Rif S. El-Mallakh, M.D.
Director, Mood Disorders Research Program
Department of Psychiatry and Behavioral Sciences
University of Louisville School of Medicine
Louisville, Kentucky

Washington, DC
London, England

Copyright © 1996 American Psychiatric Press, Inc.

ALL RIGHTS RESERVED

Manufactured in the United States of America on acid-free paper
First Edition   99 98 97 96   4 3 2 1

American Psychiatric Press, Inc.
1400 K Street, N.W., Washington, DC 20005

Library of Congress Cataloging-in-Publication Data
El-Mallakh, Rif S., 1956–   .
    Lithium : action and mechanisms / Rif S. El-Mallakh.
      p. cm. -- (Progress in psychiatry series ; #50)
    Includes bibliographical references and index.
    ISBN 0-88048-481-0 (alk. paper)
      1. Lithium—Therapeutic use.   2. Lithium—Mechanism of action.
3. Lithium—Toxicology.   I. Title.   II. Series.
      [DNLM: 1. Lithium—therapeutic use.   2. Bipolar Disorder--drug
therapy.   3. Lithium—pharmacology.   W1 PR6781L no.50 1996 / QV
77.9 E48L 1996]
RC483.5.L5E4   1996
615'.2381--dc20
DNLM/DLC
for Library of Congress   95-39522
                                                                             CIP

British Library Cataloguing in Publication Data
A CIP record is available from the British Library.

To Peggy, James, and Thomas

Contents

Introduction to the Progress in Psychiatry Series

The Progress in Psychiatry Series is designed to capture in print the excitement that comes from assembling a diverse group of experts from various locations to examine in detail the newest information about a developing aspect of psychiatry. This series emerged as a collaboration between the American Psychiatric Association's Scientific Program Committee and the American Psychiatric Press, Inc. Great interest is generated by a number of the symposia presented each year at the American Psychiatric Association annual meeting, and we realized that much of the information presented there, carefully assembled by people who are deeply immersed in a given area, would unfortunately not appear together in print. The symposia sessions at the annual meetings provide an unusual opportunity for experts who otherwise might not meet on the same platform to share their diverse viewpoints for 3 hours. Some new themes are repeatedly reinforced and gain credence, whereas in other instances disagreements emerge, enabling the audience and now the reader to reach informed decisions about new directions in the field. The Progress in Psychiatry Series allows us to publish and capture some of the best of the symposia and thus provide an in-depth treatment of specific areas that might not otherwise be presented in broader review formats.

Psychiatry is, by nature, an interface discipline, combining the study of mind and brain, of individual and social environments, of the humane and the scientific. Therefore, progress in the field is rarely linear—it often comes from unexpected sources. Furthermore, new developments emerge from an array of viewpoints that do not necessarily provide immediate agreement but rather expert examination of the issues. We intend to present innovative ideas and data that will enable you, the reader, to participate in this process.

We believe the Progress in Psychiatry Series will provide you with an opportunity to review timely information in specific fields of interest as they are developing. We hope you find that the excitement of the presentations is captured in the written word and that this book proves to be informative and enjoyable reading.

David Spiegel, M.D.
Series Editor
Progress in Psychiatry Series

Progress in Psychiatry Series Titles

Lithium: Actions and Mechanisms (#50)
By Rif S. El-Mallakh, M.D.

Role of Sexual Abuse in Etiology of Borderline Personality Disorder (#49)
Edited by Mary C. Zanarini, Ed.D.

Water Balance in Schizophrenia (#48)
Edited by David B. Schnur, M.D., and Darrell G. Kirch, M.D.

NMR Spectroscopy in Psychiatric Brain Disorders (#47)
Edited by Henry A. Nasrallah, M.D., and Jay W. Pettegrew, M.D.

Does Stress Cause Psychiatric Illness? (#46)
Edited by Carolyn M. Mazure, Ph.D.

Biological and Neurobehavioral Studies of Borderline Personality Disorder (#45)
Edited by Kenneth R. Silk, M.D.

Severe Depressive Disorders (#44)
Edited by Leon Grunhaus, M.D., and John F. Greden, M.D.

Clinical Advances in Monoamine Oxidase Inhibitor Therapies (#43)
Edited by Sidney H. Kennedy, M.D., F.R.C.P.C.

Catecholamine Function in Posttraumatic Stress Disorder: Emerging Concepts (#42)
Edited by M. Michele Murburg, M.D.

Central Nervous System Peptide Mechanisms in Stress and Depression (#30)
Edited by S. Craig Risch, M.D.

Neuropeptides and Psychiatric Disorders (#29)
Edited by Charles B. Nemeroff, M.D., Ph.D.

Negative Schizophrenic Symptoms: Pathophysiology and Clinical Implications (#28)
Edited by John F. Greden, M.D., and Rajiv Tandon, M.D.

The Neuroleptic Nonresponsive Patient: Characterization and Treatment (#27)
Edited by Burt Angrist, M.D., and S. Charles Schulz, M.D.

Combination Pharmacotherapy and Psychotherapy for Depression (#26)
Edited by Donna Manning, M.D., and Allen J. Frances, M.D.

Treatment Strategies for Refractory Depression (#25)
Edited by Steven P. Roose, M.D., and Alexander H. Glassman, M.D.

Biological Rhythms, Mood Disorders, Light Therapy, and the Pineal Gland (#24)
Edited by Mohammad Shafii, M.D., and Sharon Lee Shafii, R.N., B.S.N.

Family Environment and Borderline Personality Disorder (#23)
Edited by Paul Skevington Links, M.D.

Amino Acids in Psychiatric Disease (#22)
Edited by Mary Ann Richardson, Ph.D.

Serotonin in Major Psychiatric Disorders (#21)
Edited by Emil F. Coccaro, M.D., and Dennis L. Murphy, M.D.

Personality Disorders: New Perspectives on Diagnostic Validity (#20)
Edited by John M. Oldham, M.D.

Can Schizophrenia Be Localized in the Brain? (#6)
Edited by Nancy C. Andreasen, M.D., Ph.D.

The Psychiatric Implications of Menstruation (#5)
Edited by Judith H. Gold, M.D., F.R.C.P.C.

Post-Traumatic Stress Disorder in Children (#4)
Edited by Spencer Eth, M.D., and Robert S. Pynoos, M.D., M.P.H.

Treatment of Affective Disorders in the Elderly (#3)
Edited by Charles A. Shamoian, M.D.

Premenstrual Syndrome: Current Findings and Future Directions (#2)
Edited by Howard J. Osofsky, M.D., Ph.D., and
Susan J. Blumenthal, M.D.

The Borderline: Current Empirical Research (#1)
Edited by Thomas H. McGlashan, M.D.

Preface

Manic-depressive illness is as dualistic as its name and its course. The disease robs people of stability and calm in exchange for fleeting euphoria and energy. People with manic-depressive illness may be rewarded with creative minds yet not be given the ability or opportunity to apply that creativity. Manic-depressive illness is a flim-flam disease that cheats people out of their lives.

Lithium, a simple, light metal, has restored the lives and brought to life the dreams of an untold number of individuals with manic-depressive illness. It is certainly the simplest medicinal agent available. Its ability to alleviate the signs and symptoms of one of the most enigmatic of diseases makes it quite intriguing. This alone makes lithium compelling to study; however, many pragmatic issues make lithium essential to investigate.

Lithium is nearly as dualistic as the disease it treats. The difference between the healing powers and the destructive powers of lithium is miniscule. I begin this book by exploring both the therapeutic and toxic actions of lithium. There is no question that these are invaluable things to know about lithium if one prescribes it or consumes it. However, my purpose goes beyond immediate practical knowledge. The clinical section of this book is intended as the infrastructure on which the second portion is built.

In the basic section of the book, I examine the neurochemical and cellular consequences of lithium. I explore our current state of knowledge concerning lithium, gather disparate work onto the same pages, and integrate this into a whole that can lead to an understanding of not just lithium, but manic depression as well.

I have tried to make the book readable and understandable to a varied audience. Consequently, some readers may feel that I have been excessively simplistic, whereas others may think I have been overly complex. However, I believe the greatest number of readers will find the book both manageable and useful. Also, I hope that most will regard it as insightful and enjoyable.

Acknowledgments

M any people were instrumental in the ultimate fruition of this book. My wife and children tolerated with grace and patience my absence and my occasionally fanatical preoccupation. I am also particularly indebted to Richard Jed Wyatt, M.D., Chief, Neuropsychiatry Branch, National Institute of Mental Health, and Allan Tasman, M.D., Professor and Chairman, Department of Psychiatry and Behavioral Sciences, University of Louisville School of Medicine, for their incessant encouragement. David Spiegel, M.D., Chairman, Department of Psychiatry, University of Illinois, College of Medicine at Peoria; Neil Liebowitz, Department of Psychiatry, University of Connecticut; and Roger Meyer, M.D., Vice President for Medical Affairs and Executive Dean, George Washington University, provided formative guidance. Patrick O'Hayer, M.A. of Libertyville, Illinois, reviewed the manuscript. Work for various sections of the volume was conducted or completed while receiving financial support from the Peoria Association of Retarded Citizens, the National Alliance for Research in Schizophrenia and Depression, and the University of Louisville.

Section I

Clinical Experience

Chapter 1

Lithium in Bipolar Illness

Nearly 200 years ago, while on a mineralogical expedition to Sweden, a Brazilian scientist, Jose de Andrada, discovered two new minerals in an iron ore mine on the island of Utö. He named one mineral petalite and the other spodumene. In 1817, a Swedish chemist, Johan August Arfwedson, determined the composition of petalite and discovered that 4% contained a previously unknown alkali metal. His supervisor, the renowned Swedish chemist Baron Jons Jacob Berzelius, suggested the name lithion (F. N. Johnson 1984).

Following the 1841 observation by Dr. A. Lipowitz that lithium carbonate salts dissolve uric acid (and the subsequent popularization of that fact by Alexander Ure), lithium became a staple treatment for gout and all the ills it was believed to produce (F. N. Johnson 1984). Indeed, the fascination with lithium extended beyond the traditional medical profession, with lithiated water becoming a common cure-all and lithiated beer being brewed in Wisconsin (Jefferson 1989; Redmann and Jefferson 1985).

As interest in using lithium to treat gout was waning, a Danish internist, Carl Lange, in 1886 and again in 1897, reported that lithium salts play a therapeutic and preventive role in treating recurrent depression. Fritz Lange, Carl Lange's brother, wrote in his 1894 book, *The Most Important Groups of Insanity,* that lithium carbonate worked as an antidepressant (F. N. Johnson 1984). Unfortunately, the work of the Lange brothers remained obscure and was eventually lost. A generation would pass before the psychotropic effects of lithium would be rediscovered.

LITHIUM THERAPY IN ACUTE MANIA

John F. J. Cade, an Australian, became interested in the organic causes of mental disorders when he was a prisoner of war in World

War II. At the end of the war, he returned to his native Melbourne, where he initiated studies to search for the metabolite that was responsible for mania. Believing that uric acid might play a role in the illness, he initiated several studies with lithium salts (F. N. Johnson 1984). His observations that lithium injections produced extraordinary placidity in guinea pigs (probably a toxic manifestation) led him to believe that lithium might possess an antiexcitement property (Cade 1949). After ensuring that lithium did not produce adverse side effects by taking it himself, Cade carefully initiated his clinical studies (F. N. Johnson 1984). All 10 manic patients he initially treated showed considerable improvement; however, six schizophrenic patients and three depressive patients did not respond to treatment (Cade 1949).

Three other Australians quickly replicated Cade's original report. Noack and Trautner (1951) of the University of Melbourne reported that 25 of their 30 manic patients improved after treatment with lithium; Glesinger (1954) of Western Australia reported that 15 of 21 manic patients showed significant improvement (Table 1–1). Even so, it was a young Danish psychiatrist who was to prove to be the champion of lithium therapy. Mogens Schou was the driving force that ensured that Cade's work would not have the same fate as that of the Lange brothers.

Schou, Juel-Nielsen, Strömgren, and Voldby (1954) arranged the first double-blind, placebo-controlled study of lithium in acute mania (Table 1–1). Lithium or placebo was administered in a crossover design over 2-week periods. Unfortunately, when they published their results, the researchers combined the data derived from this blinded study with data from the open administration of lithium, and they did not apply any statistical analysis to the data (Schou et al. 1954). The first double-blind study done according to modern standards was conducted in England by Maggs (1963), and the first American study was conducted by Bunney, Goodwin, Davis, and Fawcett in 1968 and extended in 1969 (Goodwin et al. 1969) (Table 1–1). All of these studies showed a consistent picture of lithium's superiority to placebo in nearly 70% of the patients (Table 1–1), with a smaller fraction of patients obtaining good symptomatic relief. A few well-publicized studies with response rates over 80% (Goodwin and Ebert 1973; Schou 1959) created the lin-

Table 1–1. Open and controlled studies examining the efficacy of lithium therapy in acute mania

N	N Improved (%)	Comment	Study
10	10 (100)	Open	Cade 1949
30	25 (83)	Open	Noack & Trautner 1951
21	15 (71)	Open	Glesinger 1954
38	32 (84)	Partially open, partially double-blind, placebo-controlled but presented as combined	Schou et al. 1954
35	30 (86)	Open	Reviewed in F. N. Johnson 1984[a]
48	39 (81)	Open	Schou et al. 1955
10	9 (90)	Experiential	Gershon & Trautner 1956
37	34 (92)	Open	Rice 1956
14	13 (93)	Open	Andriani et al. 1958
32	24 (75)	Open	Belling 1959
119	91 (76)	Experiential	Schou 1959
25	17 (68)	Open administration, single-blind rating	Wharton & Fieve 1966
68	61 (90)	Open; some patients received other medications	Schlagerhauf et al. 1966
22	21 (95)	Open; moderately ill patients	Blinder 1968
348	159 (46)		Reviewed by Kline 1969[b]
75	55 (73)	Open	van der Velde 1970
17	16 (94)	Open	Kingstone 1960
19	13 (68)	Open	Swann et al. 1987
28		Only 18 completed the study; lithium superior to placebo	Maggs 1963
2	2 (100)	Double-blind, placebo-controlled	Bunney et al. 1968
10	7 (70)	Double-blind, placebo-controlled	Goodwin et al. 1969

(continued)

Table 1–1. Open and controlled studies examining the efficacy of lithium therapy in acute mania *(continued)*

N	N Improved (%)	Comment	Study
38	28.5(75)	Double-blind, placebo-controlled. Data analyzed for 98 manic periods. 75% of episodes responded. Improvement rate for placebo was 40.5%, $P < .05$	Stokes et al. 1971
1046	697.5(67)	TOTAL	

Note. Overall efficacy is 69%.
[a]Two French studies are reported.
[b]Data are from a wide range of studies from the Soviet Union, Czechoslovakia, Italy, and France.

gering impression that early studies had overestimated the effectiveness of lithium therapy.

Although lithium has clearly demonstrated efficacy in acute mania, that effect is maximal after 7–10 days. Consequently, in the acute setting, faster acting agents, such as neuroleptics (Kane 1988; Lenox et al. 1992; Prien et al. 1972; Rees and Davis 1965; Schou 1968) and benzodiazepines (Chouinard 1988; Lenox et al. 1992; Modell et al. 1985) are often safer than, and at least as effective as (and often more effective than), lithium.

LITHIUM PROPHYLAXIS

Although lithium was introduced into modern psychiatric practice as a treatment for acute mania, it appears to be much more effective in the prophylaxis of pathological moods in bipolar illness than in their treatment. The prophylactic effects of lithium became quickly obvious to the clinicians who prescribed it on a regular basis. However, observations regarding lithium's prophylactic action were first published by two academically inexperienced psychiatrists, G. P. Hartigan (1963) and Paul C. Baastrup (1964; F. N. Johnson 1984). Both psychiatrists had made their observations circa 1957, but their insecurity regarding the enterprise of publishing delayed the reports (F. N. Johnson 1984). Baastrup also initiated a prospective study in which he followed 88 patients who were openly administered lithium for some 6.5 years. In 1967, he published his results in collaboration with Schou. Eighty-one patients exhibited a decrease in relapse frequency (Baastrup and Schou 1967). This observation was reproduced in a larger sample of 244 patients (Angst et al. 1970).

Blackwell and Shepherd (1968), citing some methodological problems, called into question the findings of Baastrup and his colleagues and initiated a scientific debate that persisted into the early 1970s (Blackwell 1972). At the heart of this debate was the definition of future anticipated relapses (i.e., how could you prove that the patients would have indeed relapsed if they were not taking lithium?). Although this may have been a valid statistical question, the answer was obvious to the clinician. Bipolar illness was long known to have a progressively deteriorating course if left untreated. Specifically, mood shifts become much more frequent and euthymic periods decrease (Angst et al. 1969; Post 1990; Swift 1907); an interruption of this pattern quickly becomes evident.

Despite the scientific debate, the use of lithium prophylaxis spread consistently throughout most of Europe even before the outcome of double-blind trials was known (Schou 1973). In the publications concerning double-blind trials in the 1970s (Baastrup et al. 1970; Coppen et al. 1971; Cundall et al. 1972; Fieve et al. 1976; Hullin et al. 1972, 1975; Prien et al. 1973; Quitkin et al. 1978; Stallone et al. 1973), and in the more recent reports on discontinuation trials (Cordess 1982; Faedda et al. 1993; Sashidharan and McGuire 1983; Small et al. 1971a; Strober et al. 1990), lithium has repeatedly proven its prophylactic efficacy for both mania and depression in bipolar patients. Lithium treatment generally produces a greater than twofold reduction in the risk of relapse, from more than 79% in placebo-treated bipolar patients to a 34% or 36% rate in lithium-treated patients (Appleton and Davis 1980; Baldessarini 1985; J. M. Davis 1976). Over a 2-year period, 58% of bipolar patients will be protected from relapse (Melia 1970; Prien et al. 1973; Stallone et al. 1973). The issue becomes even more important if the initial reports of lithium withdrawal emergent refractoriness (Maj et al. 1995; Post 1990, 1992) are confirmed.

LITHIUM THERAPY IN RECURRENT DEPRESSION

Although the Lange brothers reported a possible antidepressant effect of lithium in the late 1800s, that fact had to be rediscovered a century later. Schou, Hartigan, Baastrup, and others noted that the prophylactic effect of lithium was not limited to the prevention of recurrent manias, but that depressions were also prevented. This fact was well appreciated by Schou, whose brother's frequently recurrent and paralyzing depressions had been banished by lithium maintenance (F. N. Johnson 1984). However, the antidepressant effect of lithium has been more difficult to confirm than its antimanic effect. This is probably because lithium is more effective in treating bipolar depression than nonbipolar depression (see Table 1–2 and Chapter 2). The response rate of 67.5% among depressed bipolar patients is quite similar to the response rate of 69% among manic patients (see Tables 1–1 and 1–2). However, among "nonbipolar" patients, the lithium response rate is only 51% (Table 1–2), which is higher than the typical placebo response rate of 20%–30% (Baldessarini 1985). Moreover, the 51% figure may be artificially inflated by bipolar II individuals or by "unrecognized" bipolar individuals (i.e., individuals who have a bipolar illness but have not as yet experienced a manic episode). If this is true, then lithium alone may be no more efficacious than placebo in nonbipolar depression.

LITHIUM NONRESPONDERS

More than 30% of manic or depressed bipolar individuals will not respond to the acute administration of lithium, and a large fraction of patients will relapse despite lithium prophylaxis. Nonresponders have generally been felt to be atypical (Baastrup and

Table 1–2. Studies examining the efficacy of lithium in the treatment
of depression, subtyped into bipolar and nonbipolar
depressions

N	N Improved (%)	Comment	Study
Bipolar patients			
8	6 (75)	Open	Hartigan 1963
7	7(100)	Open	Dyson & Mendels 1968
13	10 (77)	Controlled	Goodwin et al. 1969
18	0	Controlled. All improved on lithium but not different from placebo	Stokes et al. 1971
40	32 (80)	Controlled	Goodwin et al. 1972
6	6(100)	Controlled	Noyes et al. 1974
13	9 (69)	Controlled	Mendels 1975
9	7 (78)	Controlled	Baron et al. 1975
114	77 (68)	TOTAL	
Nonbipolar patients			
3	0	Open	Cade 1949
14	8 (57)	Open; all had previously failed electroconvulsive therapy	Reviewed in Schou 1968[a]
24	10 (42)	Open	Andriani et al. 1958
24	12 (50)	Open; 10 of the responders had "cyclothymic personality"	Dyson & Mendels 1968
5	5(100)	With placebo substitution, 3 patients relapsed; 1 had incomplete response to lithium	Noyes et al. 1971
98	53 (54)	Open	Nahunek et al. 1970

(continued)

Table 1–2.   Studies examining the efficacy of lithium in the treatment of depression, subtyped into bipolar and nonbipolar depressions *(continued)*

N	N Improved (%)	Comment	Study
Nonbipolar patients (continued)			
21		Open; all patients had incomplete response to lithium alone; some were bipolar	Himmelhoch et al. 1977b
5	2 (40)	Controlled	Goodwin et al. 1969
12	4 (33)	Controlled	Goodwin et al. 1972
10	10(100)	Controlled; 5 with only partial response	G. Johnson 1974
16	7 (44)	Controlled	Noyes et al. 1974
8	4 (50)	Controlled	Mendels 1975
14	3 (21)	Controlled	Baron et al. 1975
65	30 (46)	Total among controlled studies	
233	118 (51)	TOTAL	

[a]Vojtechovsky M, 1957, as reviewed in Schou 1968.

Schou 1967; Schou et al. 1954), to experience mixed states or dysphoric mania (Himmelhoch and Garfinkel 1986; Keller et al. 1986; Prien et al. 1988; Secunda et al. 1987), or to cycle very rapidly (Abou-Saleh and Coppen 1986; Dunner and Fieve 1974; Goodnick et al. 1987; Prien et al. 1973). Conversely, more classic or typical manic episodes and a family history of bipolar illness predict a favorable response to lithium treatment and prophylaxis in both adults (Abou-Saleh and Coppen 1986; Maj et al. 1984, 1985) and children (DeLong and Aldershof 1987). These patterns may suggest that lithium has a specific action in a biologically distinct bipolar disease, or simply that lithium can more readily control symptoms when bipolar illness is less severe (i.e., that mixed states and rapid cycling may represent a more severe manifestation of the bipolar spectrum [Post 1990]). Although this question cannot be answered adequately, it is becoming clear that some patients who are not responsive to lithium may respond to valproate (Calabrese et al. 1992; Calabrese and Delucchi 1990; McElroy et al. 1988) or clozapine (McElroy et al. 1991; Suppes et al. 1992). However, it is likely that some of the more common factors associated with lithium nonresponse may be related to suboptimal use of lithium. The frequent occurrences of relatively minor side effects in the course of lithium therapy (see Chapter 3) tend to decrease compliance with outpatient lithium regimens (Cochran 1986; Gitlin et al. 1989) or tempt clinicians to lower the dose and consequent lithium level. This may cause a dramatic increase in relapse rates (Gelenberg et al. 1989) or subsyndromal symptoms, which may suggest incomplete response (Keller et al. 1992). There is an unfortunate dearth of attempts to maximize lithium's beneficial actions while reducing its toxic potential and bothersome side effects.

However, one such promising avenue, which, unfortunately, is still not widely employed, is the determination of intraerythrocyte lithium levels or lithium ratios (El-Mallakh 1994) (also see Chapter 6). Some (Casper et al. 1976; Cazzullo et al. 1975; Flemenbaum et al. 1978; Maj et al. 1984; Mendels et al. 1976; Sacchetti et al. 1977; Yassa and Nair 1985) have argued that although not universally accepted (Knorring et al. 1976; Rybakowski and Strzyzewski 1976), the likelihood of a therapeutic response to lithium can be predicted by the lithium ratio (usually defined as intraerythrocyte lithium levels/plasma lithium level). Specifically, lithium ratios of < 0.4 are associated with refractoriness to lithium, whereas those ratios of > 0.4 are associated with high response rates. Similarly, higher lithium ratios or higher intraerythrocyte lithium levels are associated with side effects (such as tremor, polyuria, and polydipsia) (Albrect and Müller-Oerlinghausen 1976; Hewick and Murray 1976) and abnormal electroencephalograms (EEGs) (Zakowska-Dabrowska and Rybakowski 1973). If the site of action of lithium is intracellular, as is widely believed (see Section II), then one may argue that lithium response is related to the accumulation of therapeutic intracellular lithium levels, perhaps independently of serum levels. Consequently, it would seem worthwhile to attempt to define the therapeutic range of lithium ratios or intraerythrocyte lithium levels (El-Mallakh 1994).

CONCLUSIONS AND IMPLICATIONS

The data reveal that lithium therapy can be of unequivocal benefit in the treatment of acutely ill bipolar patients and in the prophylaxis of pathological moods in bipolar illness. It also appears that unipolar patients get minimal benefit from lithium alone, although these findings are disputed (see Chapter 2). Lithium has undoubtedly reduced suffering and misery in a large number of individuals. Lithium extended the average life span of a woman with a typical bipolar illness type of by 6.5 years, reestablished 10 years of otherwise lost life activity, and eliminated 8.5 years of medical and psychiatric health complications (Gelenberg 1988). This benefit translates into a savings of approximately $400 million annually in the United States alone (Reifman and Wyatt 1980). It would seem that even greater treasures lie in deciphering lithium's mechanism of action.

Chapter 2

Utility of Lithium in Other Conditions

The initial, and generally unexpected, success of lithium in the management of bipolar illness spawned the hope that lithium might be beneficial in a variety of other psychiatric and neurological conditions. Because of the wide diversity of diseases for which lithium therapy has been attempted, one might conclude that decisions to administer lithium were arrived at randomly; however, this would be erroneous. In every case, lithium trials were initiated on the basis of animal data or serendipitous clinical observations. Unfortunately, lithium has proven to be a somewhat limited agent, with superior efficacy only in mood disorders. In this chapter, I review some of the work done with nonbipolar illnesses.

UNIPOLAR DEPRESSION

The discovery and documentation of the therapeutic and prophylactic efficacy of lithium in bipolar illness understandably generated much excitement and enthusiasm. In particular, lithium's usefulness in treating bipolar depression created hope that lithium might also be useful in the treatment and prevention of recurrent episodes of unipolar depression. However, the experimental evidence has not been overwhelming. When administered as the sole agent, lithium is effective in 45% of unipolar patients (see Table 1–2). In studies comparing lithium with tricyclic antidepressants (each as the sole agent), and in studies of populations of mixed bipolar and unipolar depression (Mendels et al. 1972b; Watanabe et al. 1975; Worrall et al. 1979) and of homogenous unipolar depression (Khan 1981), lithium was equivalent to tricyclic antidepressants in the treatment of acute depression. In the prevention of depressive relapse, lithium was equivalent to (Glen et al. 1984) or inferior to (Prien et al 1984) a tricyclic antidepressant regimen. If the potential for lithium toxicity and side effects is factored into the analysis (see Chapter 3), lithium becomes a significantly inferior agent for unipolar depression.

Where lithium has shown unquestioned efficacy is in the augmentation of standard antidepressant therapy in poorly responsive patients. Following the original uncontrolled report in 1968 by Zall and colleagues, several investigators combined lithium and antidepressant therapy in an attempt to cure treatment-resistant depression. To date, more than 50 reports of lithium augmentation have been published. With minor exceptions (e.g., Heninger et al. 1983; Kantor et al. 1982; Zusky et al. 1988), they all present similar results (e.g., dé Montigny et al. 1981, 1983, 1985; Himmelhoch et al. 1972; Joffe et al. 1993; Lingjaerde et al. 1974; Louie and Meltzer 1984; Nelson and Mazure 1986; Pope et al. 1988; Price et al. 1983, 1985, 1986; Thase et al. 1989). Generally, more than half of the individuals not responding to sole agent antidepressant treatment administered for over 4 weeks improved within 1–4 weeks of adding lithium to the regimen. There may be no relationship between lithium levels and response (dé Montigny et al. 1983; Heninger et al. 1983), or lower lithium levels may actually be more beneficial (dé Montigny et al. 1985; Fontaine et al. 1991; Madakasira 1986). Interestingly, a significant fraction of patients experienced only transient improvement (Heninger et al. 1983; Kantor et al. 1982; Louie and Meltzer 1984). This seems to be even more the case in some placebo-controlled studies (Heninger et al. 1983; Kantor et al. 1982; Zusky et al. 1988). If this is true, the mechanism by which lithium augments antidepressant medications in unipolar depression may be different from the mechanism of treatment and prophylaxis of abnormal moods in bipolar illness—where the effect may last a lifetime.

SCHIZOAFFECTIVE ILLNESS

A significant fraction of patients exhibit mood symptoms and chronic psychoses superimposed over a chronic, generally deteriorating course. The level of functioning and the prognosis of these patients is generally worse than in bipolar illness but better than in schizophrenia (Samson et al. 1988). In North America, these patients are frequently diagnosed with schizoaffective illness (Procci 1976), whereas in Europe, they are likely to be diagnosed as having a cycloid psychotic disorder (Perris 1988). Unfortunately, the diagnostic criteria for schizoaffective illness are quite vague (American Psychiatric Association 1994), and the validity of the diagnostic category is itself questioned (Pope et al. 1980). A significant number of investigators believe that most individuals diagnosed with schizoaffective disorder are either severely affected bipolar or mildly affected schizophrenic patients. Despite these basic problems, psychopharmacological investigations have been attempted in this group.

Delva and Letemerdia (1982) performed a critical review of the literature between 1951 and 1980. Nearly all investigations studied the prophylactic effects of lithium in schizoaffective illness. Delva and Letemerdia found 113 patients reported in 19 publications, including case presentations and open and controlled studies. Overall, 82% of the patients showed a favorable response to lithium (Delva and Letemerdia 1982). However, when anecdotal reports are excluded, the response rate drops to 75%, and when uncontrolled studies are excluded, the response rate drops to 40%. Unfortunately, many of these studies had a wide variety of methodological problems, including a generally minute sample size (average of six patients per study; if case reports are excluded, the average is 7.7 patients per study) (Delva and Letemerdia 1982) and treatment outcome that was evaluated when patients had demonstrated toxic plasma lithium levels (up to 2.55 mEq/L) (G. Johnson et al. 1968).

More recent efforts to answer the question have not been any more enlightening. One of the most thoughtful studies was conducted by Maj (1984, 1988). He diagnosed the subjects by a variety of different diagnostic systems and followed 48 patients for 2 years to determine whether open administration of lithium was effective in schizoaffective illness and, if so, what characteristics are associated with efficacy. Lithium therapy resulted in a significant decrease in total episodes (compared with those prior to the initiation of lithium, $P < .001$) and total psychiatric morbidity ($P < .01$).

However, the only predictor of response was a previous history consistent with a diagnosis of bipolar illness; patients with a predominantly schizophrenic or schizodepressive schizoaffective illness did not benefit (Maj 1988).

SCHIZOPHRENIA

There is a great degree of symptomatic overlap between acutely ill schizophrenic patients and acutely manic bipolar patients. Therefore, it was a logical step to attempt to treat acute schizophrenic exacerbations with lithium. Cade did so in 1949 and found that the symptoms of agitation and motoric hyperactivity decreased in three of six patients. Subsequent open studies revealed strikingly similar results. Sixty percent of 269 schizophrenic patients treated openly with lithium before 1960 showed some improvement (reviewed in Gershon and Yuwiler 1960). In nearly all the cases, the improvement was limited to the level of psychomotor activity (Gershon and Yuwiler 1960).

Placebo-controlled studies have generally found similar results. As a sole agent in the control of acute schizophrenic psychosis, lithium is probably superior to placebo but inferior to neuroleptic medications (P. E. Alexander et al. 1979; Garver et al. 1984; Shopsin et al. 1971b). When lithium shows efficacy, it is usually related to the presence of active mood symptoms, previous mood episodes, or a family history of therapeutic response to lithium therapy (Sautter et al. 1990) or affective disorder (Atre-Vaidya and Taylor 1989).

When combined with neuroleptic agents, lithium appears to potentiate the antipsychotic action of the drugs (Carman et al. 1981; Growe et al. 1979; Lewis et al. 1986; Small et al. 1975). This effect is reminiscent of the one seen in acute unipolar depression (see above) and delusional depression (Nelson and Mazure 1986; Price et al. 1983). However, the transient nature of the response in depression has not been reported in schizophrenia.

When this phenomenon is investigated further, a subgroup of patients diagnosed as schizophrenic and exhibiting a generally stable level of interepisode functioning (occasionally labeled "good prognosis" schizophrenia patients) appear to be the ones who benefit from lithium therapy (Hirschowitz et al. 1980; Sautter and

Garver 1985). Some authors believe that these so-called lithium-responsive schizophrenic patients may actually have a variant affective disorder (Sautter and Garver 1985).

ALCOHOLISM

Affective illness has a high prevalence of comorbidity with alcoholism, although the rate of comorbidity may not be as high as originally believed (Kranzler and Liebowitz 1988; Weissman et al. 1980). This long-recognized association prompted Kline et al. (1974) to test the efficacy of lithium in preventing alcohol abuse relapse. Lithium significantly reduced both readmission rates and episodes of relapse when compared with placebo in depressed alcoholic patients (Kline et al. 1974). More recently, another double-blind, placebo-controlled lithium trial in nondepressed alcoholic patients revealed a 67% abstinence rate among patients with therapeutic lithium levels compared with a rate of < 44% for noncompliant or poorly compliant patients (Fawcett et al. 1987). Although these effects on abstinence were independent of any effect on mood or social withdrawal (Fawcett et al. 1987; Kline et al. 1974), the project design in the latter study (i.e., examining compliance with abstinence as a function of compliance with medication) prevents any useful conclusions. Compliance with medication may simply be a measure of individual motivation. In a recently published prospective double-blind, placebo-controlled study, there was no demonstrable effect of lithium on abstinence even in depressed patients (de la Fuente et al. 1989).

MISCELLANEOUS PSYCHIATRIC CONDITIONS

In addition to these well-studied uses, lithium has been recommended or tried in a variety of other psychiatric conditions. For example, aggressive behavior is a symptom common to a wide range of psychiatric and neurological disorders. In anecdotal, open, and a few controlled studies, lithium has been found to have a general anti-aggressive effect. Because most aggressive acts are impulsive, this effect may also be viewed as an anti-impulsive property.

Lithium may reduce aggression in adults with documented central nervous system pathology (Hale and Donaldson 1982; Leonard et al. 1974; Mehta 1976; Rosenbaum and Barry 1975; Sheard et al. 1976; Worrall 1974) and in adults without it (Rifkin et al. 1972; Tupin et al. 1973). However, most authors believe that lithium is useful in this setting only when a significant affective component coexists (Greenhill et al. 1973; Hale and Donaldson 1982; Kerbeshian et al. 1987; Youngerman and Canino 1978).

With respect to children, researchers who conducted open and controlled studies reported that lithium is useful in controlling aggression, the impulsivity of conduct disorder (Platt et al. 1984), and attention deficit hyperactivity disorder (R. P. Brown et al. 1983; Whitehead and Clark 1970). Lithium has also been found to be useful in treating brain-damaged children (Campbell and Spencer 1988; Luchins and Kojka 1989). Although Campbell , Platt, and collegues have not found a concomitant mood component in lithium-responsive children (Platt et al. 1984), the diagnosis of mood disorders (in general) and bipolar illness (in particular) in children is difficult and controversial (Weller et al. 1986). Furthermore, several reports suggest that bipolar illness in children may be misdiagnosed as either conduct disorder (Carlson and Kashani 1988; Issac 1992; Kutcher et al. 1989; Myers et al. 1993; S. M. Schneider et al., unpublished data, 1995) or, to a lesser degree, attention deficit hyperactivity disorder (Dvoredsky and Stewart 1981; Feinstein and Wolpert 1973; Issac 1991; Reiss 1985; S. M. Schneider et al., unpublished data, 1995; Versamis and MacDonald 1972; Weinberg and Brumbach 1976).

In a late luteal phase dysphoric disorder (premenstrual tension syndromes or PMS), where placebo response can be 40%–50% (O'Brien 1982), open, controlled trials showed that lithium was helpful (O'Brien 1982; Sletten and Gershon 1966), but blind, placebo-controlled studies showed no difference between placebo and lithium (Mattsson and Schoultz 1974; K. Singer et al. 1974; Steiner et al. 1980).

SUMMARY OF PSYCHIATRIC APPLICATIONS

Although Schou's early assertion that lithium may be a mood-specific agent (1963b) is certainly debatable, a careful review of the literature suggests that there is a dearth of lithium-responsive non-

mood disorders. With the exception of its augmentation properties (where the effect may be transient), lithium utility may be
limited to patients with bipolar disorder or at least bipolar symptomatology. Recognizing this limitation is an important point in any
attempt to understand possible mechanisms of action. A limitation of lithium's action suggests that it may operate in a very specific way (or on several specific sites) to induce its therapeutic and
prophylactic effect. Subsequent discussions of mechanistic actions
will assume a unique action on bipolar illness or symptomatology.
Although this point is debatable, there is considerable evidence in
the literature to warrant this approach.

LITHIUM IN NONPSYCHIATRIC APPLICATIONS

Lithium in Neurology

Headaches.   The only well-established indication for lithium in
neurology is for cluster headache prophylaxis (L. Kudrow 1977; W.
Kudrow 1980). The prophylactic effect in most patients is maintained
with chronic treatment, when lithium is administered at affective
disorder dosages and serum levels (L. Kudrow 1977; W. Kudrow
1980). This effect is limited to cluster headaches; lithium may actually exacerbate migraine headaches (Peatfield and Rose 1981).

Movement disorders.   Animal studies have shown that concomitant chronic lithium treatment prevents the development of chronic
neuroleptic-induced dopamine receptor supersensitivity (see Chapter 4) (Gallager et al. 1978; Pert et al. 1978). This finding suggests
that lithium may be of use in hyperkinetic disorders. However,
early favorable anecdotal and open trials using lithium to control
abnormal movements in Huntington's chorea (Dalen 1973; Mattsson 1973; Manyam and Bravo-Fernandez 1973) were not confirmed
in double-blind studies (Arminoff and Marshall 1974; Leonard et
al. 1974). Likewise, early open trials of lithium in tardive dyskinesia
that showed marked improvement in abnormal movements (Dalen
1973; Reda et al. 1974, 1975; Simpson 1973) were not confirmed by
double-blind studies (Gerlach et al. 1975; Mackay et al. 1980). However, initial anecdotal reports that lithium may ameliorate the

"on–off" L-dopa syndrome of Parkinson's disease (Ross et al. 1981) appear to have been confirmed in a small, blinded, controlled study (Coffey et al. 1982). Furthermore, as might be expected from the initial murine studies (Gallager et al. 1978; Pert et al. 1978; see Chapter 4), patients who receive both lithium and neuroleptic agents chronically may be partially protected from developing tardive dyskinesia (Mukherjee et al. 1986; Waddington and Youssef 1988).

Seizures.   At toxic doses, lithium is a convulsant, producing seizures in nearly 25% of patients with severe (grade III) toxicity (El-Mallakh 1986a). However, at therapeutic doses, lithium has been hypothesized to be an anticonvulsant (El-Mallakh 1983a, 1983b), and, in the 1800s, lithium was prescribed as an antiepileptic. Indeed, in safety studies in epileptic bipolar patients, lithium has demonstrated a protective effect, showing a reduction in seizure frequency (Erwin et al. 1973; Shukla et al. 1988).

Lithium in Hematology

Leukocytes.   Psychiatrists noted early that their patients receiving lithium exhibited a mild, innocuous leukocytosis (Murphy et al. 1971b; Shopsin et al. 1971a). The realization that this represented a real increase in the granulocyte pool (Rothstein et al. 1978; Tisman et al. 1973) and that it persisted over the years of lithium administration (Pi et al. 1983) led to clinical trials. Anecdotal reports in idiopathic or heritable neutropenia have been variable (Barrett et al. 1977, 1979; Gupta et al. 1976). However, when lithium is administered during anticipated chemotherapy-induced nadir periods, there is a significant increase in granulocyte counts (Greco and Brereton 1977; Stein et al. 1977). Although some studies questioned the significance of this effect (Stein et al. 1979), most researchers found that lithium treatment reduced infections, the length of hospitalization, and antibiotic use (Collado et al. 1988; Lyman et al. 1980). Similarly, lithium reverses azidothymidine (AZT)-induced neutropenia in patients with acquired immunodeficiency syndrome (AIDS) (Roberts et al. 1988), but the significance of this finding remains to be assessed. Psychiatrists occasionally make use of the granulocyte-stimulating effect of lithium to counter the leukoleptic effect of carbamazepine while potentially boosting the antimanic actions (Brewenton 1986; Servant et al. 1988).

Platelets.   Likewise, some studies (Joffe et al. 1984; Richman et al. 1984), but not all, have reported a beneficial effect on platelet counts in patients treated with chemotherapy.

Viruses.   Lithium has also demonstrated efficacy in reducing outbreaks of recurrent labial herpes infections (Lieb 1979; Rybakowski and Amsterdam 1991). Similar effects can also be achieved with a topical application of lithium succinate (Skinner 1983). These open observations achieved partial confirmation in a double-blind, placebo-controlled study involving only one patient (Parks et al. 1988), in which a statistically significant reduction in herpes eruptions occurred while on lithium prophylaxis. This effect may be mediated, in part, by the nonspecific stimulation of granulocytosis, but lithium may also have a direct virus-replication-inhibitory action (Hartley 1983; Skinner et al. 1980).

Miscellaneous Uses in Medicine

Thyroid.   Lithium produces hypothyroidism in perhaps 3% of patients (Mannisto 1980), and elevated thyroid-stimulating hormone (TSH) may occur in 10%–20% of patients treated with lithium (Lindstedt et al. 1977; Mannisto 1980; Transbol et al. 1978). Consequently, lithium was tried in hyperthyroidism and found to be marginally effective (Hedley et al. 1978).

Diabetes.   Lithium also exerts an antidiabetic effect (Saran 1982; van der Velde and Gordon 1969; Weiss 1924). This action may be related to decreased levels of intracellular calcium, which antagonizes glucagon (El-Mallakh 1983b, 1986b). This effect is significant in diabetic patients being treated with lithium and may necessitate a reduction in the dosage of insulin or other hypoglycemic agent.

Finally, lithium has been used in the treatment of a variety of other medical disorders, including the syndrome of inappropriate antidiuretic hormone secretion, periodic paralysis, Ménière's disease, spasmodic torticollis, ulcerative colitis, and vitiligo (Lewis 1982; Schou 1979; Suwana 1975). However, reports of these uses are often anecdotal or contradictory; to date, the efficacy of lithium therapy has not been confirmed in treating these disorders.

SUMMARY OF MEDICAL EFFECTS

Lithium produces unexpected effects on such diverse conditions as neutropenia, viral infections, headaches, movement disorders, and endocrine changes. There has been minimal exploration of mechanisms by which lithium may cause these effects. In the subsequent discussion of mechanisms (Section II), I will not consider the medical consequences of lithium directly. Please note, however, that the mechanistic discussions assume that peripheral and non-neuronal tissues function in essentially the same manner. Consequently, it is believed (but will not be investigated) that the medical effects of lithium probably result from the same perbutations of cellular physiology as those that occur in the central nervous system.

Chapter 3

Lithium Toxicity

Despite its documented utility, the toxic potential of lithium limits its use. American physicians, in particular, are quite cautious. This caution stems from clinical experience in the 1940s when American cardiologists recommended using lithium chloride as a sodium chloride substitute on food. Unfortunately, the combination of excessive, uncontrolled lithium consumption, sodium restriction, and diuretic-induced sodium depletion in these cardiac patients resulted in a multitude of lithium-toxicity–related deaths (Cocoran et al. 1949; El-Mallakh 1986a). This experience produced a lasting discomfort among American physicians regarding lithium use, which is currently reflected by the fact that lithium is the only psychotropic agent that is prescribed most frequently by psychiatrists as opposed to primary care practitioners (Beardsley et al. 1988). Despite appropriate precautions, the potential of lithium toxicity continues to be a significant concern.

Acute lithium toxicity almost always has central nervous system (CNS) manifestations and is usually accompanied by increased serum lithium levels (El-Mallakh 1986a). Conversely, chronic toxic side effects are seen in a multitude of other systems and occur at therapeutic levels. In this chapter, I consider acute neurotoxicity and chronic cardiac, renal, and endocrine manifestations, as well as other toxic manifestations.

LITHIUM PHARMACOLOGY

In the United States, lithium is available as a dibasic carbonate salt in both regular and slow-release tablets and capsules. It is also avail-

---

A portion of the text is adapted from El-Mallakh 1990b. Used with permission.

able in a liquid as a citrate salt. Generally, dosages vary from 150 mg (4.06 mEq) to more than 2 g (56.84 mEq) daily, depending on renal function. Lithium is excreted primarily by the kidney, with trace amounts being lost in the saliva, sweat, and gut. Lithium has a long half-life (range 8–32 hours, mean 20–26 hours [Amdisen 1973; Groth et al. 1974; Swartz and Wilcox 1984]). Because of this factor, and because of the differential rates of transmembrane lithium transport (El-Mallakh 1983b), it takes 6–10 days for lithium to reach steady state distribution (Jenner and Lee 1976; Mendels and Frazer 1973). Theoretically, the entire daily dose can be given at one time. However, lithium is rapidly absorbed from the gut after an oral dose (Schou 1957) and reaches peak serum levels within 3 hours (Baldessarini and Lipinski 1975). This rapid rise in serum lithium levels produces signs and symptoms of mild toxicity (Beardsley et al. 1988; El-Mallakh 1984). Consequently, single, large doses of lithium are frequently poorly tolerated. Lithium is best administered in two to three daily doses with meals or once at bedtime using slow-release formulations.

Lithium has a narrow therapeutic index. Generally, therapeutic serum lithium levels are held to be between .5 and 1.2 mEq/L, and levels above 1.5 mEq/L are considered to be in the toxic range (El-Mallakh 1986a). Individual variation makes these numbers general guidelines only.

Several investigators have recommended protocols that predict the lithium dosage needed to achieve steady-state therapeutic levels (Cooper et al. 1973; Coppen et al. 1966; Gengo et al. 1973; P. J. Perry et al. 1986). Most of these protocols advocate the use of a single lithium level 24 hours after a 600-mg test dose to predict the appropriate dosage. Although these studies report a high degree of accuracy in predicting dosage requirements, there are several reasons for following a more conservative approach, particularly in the acutely ill patient. First, it should be remembered that lithium toxicity occurs most frequently within the first 2 weeks after initiation of therapy or an increase of dosage (El-Mallakh 1986a). This toxicity is partially a result of the observation that calculated lithium half-lives lengthen as steady state is approached, even though dosage may not have been modified. Second, because acutely manic patients retain sodium (Coppen et al. 1966; El-Mallakh 1983a; Naylor et al. 1970), which delays the intracellular accumulation of lithium (El-Mallakh 1983b; Mendels and Frazer 1973; Mendels et al. 1976), there has been a general impression that acutely manic patients require a higher dosage of lithium. Although this belief is probably accurate, it can lead to the overmedicating of acutely ill patients. This point is further emphasized by observations that although lithium is the agent of choice in the prophylaxis of recurrent affective illness (see Chapter 1), it is equal or inferior to neuroleptic agents and electroconvulsive therapy in the acute setting (Goodwin and Zis 1979; Small et al. 1988). All of these findings suggest that caution with lithium in an acutely ill patient is preferable to aggressive treatment with lithium.

THE "PRETOXIC STATE"

Gastrointestinal upsets, consisting of diarrhea, nausea, vomiting, anorexia, mild generalized weakness, and a fine postural tremor, are fairly common in people on maintenance lithium therapy (Table 3–1). The tremor may aggravate cogwheeling in patients receiving concomitant neuroleptic agents. These symptoms are often accentuated during the absorptive rise of lithium (W. T. Brown 1976) and are thus potentially useful indicators of increasing lithium levels (El-Mallakh 1990b). As such, they may be seen to occur at serum levels < 1.0 mEq/L, are common in the first few days of the initiation of lithium therapy, and are generally more pronounced in the first few hours after an oral dose (Brown 1976; El-Mallakh 1986a). Dietary potassium supplementation (16–20 mEq/day) may ameliorate some of the troubling side effects (M. A. Cummings et al. 1988; Klemfuss, unpublished data, 1991). When these symptoms occur in a patient who previously has not been experiencing side effects, they should be considered prodromal to more severe toxicity (Table 3–1) (El-Mallakh 1984, 1986a). The most appropriate immediate measure would be to search for and treat precipitating factors, closely monitoring lithium levels and possibly decrease the lithium dose. Depending on the precipitant and general physiological state of the patient, lithium toxicity may progress over hours or a few days (El-Mallakh 1984, 1986a).

Table 3–1.   Grades of lithium toxicity

Grade	Sign or symptoms
Pretoxic state	Fine tremor
	Nausea/vomiting
	Diarrhea
	Anorexia
	Weakness
Mild (Grade I)	Drowsiness and apathy
	Blunting of affect
	Agitation or mania-like state
	Hyperreflexia, hypertonia
	Muscle fasciculations
	Dysarthria
	Ataxia
Moderate (Grade II)	Impaired consciousness
	Coarse tremor
	Pronounced ataxia
	Coarse fasciculations
	Myoclonus
	Paresis, paralysis
	Choreoathetoid movements
Severe (Grade III)	Coma or stupor
	Seizures (generalized, focal, or electroencephalogram)
	Muscle group twitching
	Spasticity
Resolution (recovery)	Ataxia
	Dysarthria
	Hyper- or hyporeflexia
	Nystagmus
	Tremor
	Spasticity
	Hypotonia

Source.   Adapted from El-Mallakh 1986a, 1990b; H. E. Hansen and Amdisen 1978.

Monitoring serum lithium levels is always recommended and is valuable. For example, maximal serum lithium levels are somewhat predictive of the outcome of toxicity (Table 3–2). However, one needs to be aware of the limitations of serum lithium values. Cases of severe lithium toxicity at therapeutic serum levels (El-Mallakh 1986a) and lack of toxic manifestations at otherwise fatal serum levels (as high as 4.5 mEq/L; see Wolpert 1977) have been reported. It is wisest to follow the clinical course and use lithium levels as supportive data. Clinical monitoring is best done by following CNS status because more than 95% of patients with toxic levels present with neurological signs and symptoms (Table 3–1).

ACUTE LITHIUM NEUROTOXICITY

The severity of lithium toxicity is marked by progressive CNS impairment (Table 3–1). Cortical depression is manifested by apathy and drowsiness, which progress to lethargy and impaired consciousness and ultimately to stupor, coma, and death (Table 3–1) (El-Mallakh 1986a). Upper motor neuron toxicity is seen clinically as hypertonia and hyperreflexia, progressing to muscle rigidity and myoclonus and finally to spasticity (Table 3–1) (El-Mallakh 1986a). Cerebellar dysfunction is seen as progressively worsening ataxia, dysmetria, and dysarthria. The peripheral neuromuscular system exhibits tremor and fasciculations (Table 3–1) (El-Mallakh 1986a). General loss of CNS homeostasis may produce various speech disturbances (Donaldson et al. 1981; G. F. Johnson 1976), focal paresis or paralysis (El-Mallakh 1986a), choreoathetoid movements (Peters 1949; Zorumski and Bakris 1983), transient cognitive deterioration (El-Mallakh and Lee 1987), or seizures (Table 3–1) (El-Mallakh 1986a; El-Mallakh and Lee 1987). Occasionally, mild lithium toxicity may produce agitation or mania-like symptoms (Table 3–1) (El-Mallakh et al. 1987). Focal lithium toxicity may also occur. In a fraction of patients undergoing concurrent electroconvulsive therapy, lithium could cause isolated cerebral toxicity without cerebellar or neuromuscular involvement (El-Mallakh 1988). In these cases, the lithium level increases intracellularly in the cerebrum secondary to the induced seizure. Serum lithium levels do not increase and may actually fall (El-Mallakh 1988).

Table 3–2. A detailed summary of cases in which sequelae were reported

Patient age & sex	Follow-up period	Sequelae	Maximum lithium level (mEq/L)	Treatment
66 M	2 months	Ataxia Dysarthria Tremor	2.4	Supportive
51 F	1 month	Slight ataxia Dysarthria Intention tremor	4.5	Supportive, sodium
36 M	6 months	Ataxia Dysarthria Intention tremor	7.6	Supportive, IV fluids, mannitol
38 F		Ataxia Dysarthria Bilateral dysdiadochokinesis Hyperreflexia Nystagmus	5.6	Forced diuresis
50 F	1 year	Ataxia Flapping tremor Choreoathetoid movements Pursing of lips	5.0	Peritoneal dialysis followed by hemodialysis
53 F	6 months	Ataxia Rhythmic tremor Choreoathetoid movements Hyperreflexia	2.3	Hemodialysis on 4th day postadmission

			7.0 (approximation)	Furosemide
28 M		Ataxia		
		Intention tremor		
		Dysmetria		
		Hyperreflexia		
34 F	6 months	Ataxia	—	Supportive
		Dysmetria		
		Nystagmus		
		Equilibrium problems		
55 F	3 years	Ataxia	2.9	—
39 M	3 weeks	Intention tremor	6.2	—
		Difficulty concentrating		
		Decrease in recent memory		
56 M	6 months	Ataxia only	—	IV fluids, delayed hemodialysis
	3 months	Dysarthria		
		Vertical nystagmus		
		Weakness		
		Hyporeflexia (lower limbs)		
		Decreased vibratory sense (lower limbs)		
56 M	3 months	Nerve conduction velocity slowed		
		Biopsy: muscle denervation		
18 F	2 months	Peripheral neuropathy on electromyogram	0.75	Supportive

(continued)

Table 3–2. A detailed summary of cases in which sequelae were reported *(continued)*

Patient age & sex	Follow-up period	Sequelae	Maximum lithium level (mEq/L)	Treatment
26 M	6 months	Fine tremor	1.2	Supportive, IV fluids
	2 years	None		
57 M	2 months	Dysarthria	2.02	Supportive
		Dextroaccented reflexes		
		Intention tremor		
M	6 months	Dysarthria	4.8	Furosemide
		Spasticity		
		Short-term memory impaired		
		Reasoning impaired		
59 M	3 months	Fine tremor	2.2	Supportive, IV fluids
62 F	7 months	Organic brain syndrome		Supportive
58 F	Few days	Organic brain syndrome	.26	Supportive
52 F	2 weeks	Decreased intellect	3.0	Supportive
33 F	—	Apathy	3.57	Supportive
62 F	1 month	Muscle weakness	2.69	
		Areflexia		
		Clinical signs of hypothyroidism		
	1 year	None		
38 M	1.5 years	Ataxia, dysmetria	5.7	Hemodialysis
		Choreoathetoid movements		

50 F	4 years	Poor short-term memory Nystagmus Ataxia, dysmetria Lead pipe rigidity Nystagmus Poor short-term memory	2.8	Hydration
31 M	1 year	Severe peripheral neuropathy Organic brain syndrome Intention tremor Dysarthria	3.63 —	Hemodialysis
38 M	10 months	Ataxia, dysmetria Dysarthria Hyperreflexia	1.6	Hemodialysis
50 F	2 years	Ataxia, upgaze palsy Hyperreflexia	3.0	Forced diuresis

Summary of Table 3–2 ($n = 27$)

Sign	Frequency (%)
Ataxia	12 (50.0)
Tremor	11 (45.8)
Dysarthria	9 (37.5)
Dementia	6 (25.0)
Dysmetria	4 (16.7)

Source. El-Mallakh 1986a.

H. E. Hansen and Amdisen (1978) proposed a gradation of lithium toxicity to evaluate severity and outcome. In their system, mild toxicity (Grade I, Table 3–1) is manifested by the earliest signs of CNS depression. Patients uneducated in the side effects of lithium rarely report these problems to their physicians because the problems are generally not severe enough for patients to seek immediate medical attention. If lithium intake is maintained, the patient may progress to moderate toxicity in a period of 1–4 days (El-Mallakh 1986a). The hallmark of moderate toxicity (Grade II, Table 3–1) is impaired consciousness. Although medical care is frequently sought at this point, progression to severe toxicity (Grade III, Table 3–1) may occur over minutes or hours.

During the acute episode of lithium neurotoxicity, the electroencephalogram (EEG) is invariably abnormal (El-Mallakh 1986a). The great majority of reports note a slowing and disorganization of electrical activity (Figure 3–1). Spiking activity is occasionally noted but only when severe toxicity is clinically evident (El-Mallakh 1986a). EEGs of neonates born to lithium-toxic mothers are always reported as normal for age (Piton et al. 1973; Wilbanks et al. 1970).

The recovery phase of acute toxicity is rarely discussed in the literature (El-Mallakh 1986a). Generally, signs and symptoms resolve gradually over a few days. With recovery from more severe toxicity, the patient may progress through the same phases of toxicity in reverse. Consequently, there may be ataxia, dysarthria, dysmetria, hyperreflexia, spasticity, or hypotonia (Table 3–1) (El-Mallakh 1986a).

Sequelae to toxicity may be persistent or permanent. Of 78 cases of acute toxicity in which some follow-up is reported, 26 patients suffered some sequelae, noted 2 weeks to 4 years later (Table 3–2) (El-Mallakh 1986a). Persistent ataxia and tremor were by far the most common sequelae (Table 3–2). Other findings, such as "organic brain syndrome" (i.e., dementia), dysarthria, hyperreflexia, and dysmetria, occurred infrequently (El-Mallakh 1986a); their significance is occasionally disputed (Goldney and Spence 1986). Choreoathetoid movements seen transiently in mild toxicity (Peters 1949; Reed et al. 1989; Zorumski and Bakris 1983) can become permanent when associated with severe toxicity (Pamphlet and Mackenzie 1982; Reed et al. 1989). Seizures occurred frequently in severe toxicity (Table 3–1), but a persistent acquired seizure disorder is quite rare (El-Mallakh and Lee 1987). Sequelae tended to occur in more severe cases (Table 3–3) or in cases in which optimal treatment was not undertaken or was delayed (Table 3–4).

Death as the outcome of acute lithium toxicity occurred in 15 of 193 cases reported in the literature (7.8%) (El-Mallakh 1986a). Death was most likely to occur when toxicity was severe (Table 3–3) or when treatment was purely supportive (11.4%) (Table 3–4); death was least likely to occur when hemodialysis was undertaken (5%) (Table 3–4) (El-Mallakh 1986a). The most frequent causes of death are circulatory collapse or respiratory failure. The observation that lithium, even at therapeutic levels, can blunt respiratory drive in the face of increased airway resistance (Weiner et al. 1983) suggests a contributing factor in terminal respiratory failure. Death as an outcome of acute toxicity was equally distributed through age and gender (El-Mallakh 1986a).

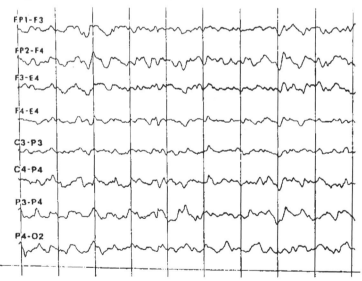

Figure 3–1. Typical slowing of EEG during severe lithium toxicity. Patient was a 52-year-old woman who took an unknown amount of lithium in a suicide attempt. Maximum lithium level was 3.2 mEq/L (Distance between lines = 1 second).

Table 3–3. Average of maximum reported serum lithium levels and outcome of acute lithium toxicity

	Death (n = 14)	Recovery with sequelae (n = 22)	Total recovery (n = 53)
Maximum serum lithium level (mEq/L)	4.24	3.26	2.54

Source. Reprinted from El-Mallakh 1986a, 1990b. Used with permission.

Table 3–4. The effect of different modes of treatment on the outcome of acute lithium toxicity (n = 188)

Treatment	Recovery*	Recovery with sequelae	Death	Total
Hemodialysis	34 (85%)**	4 (10%)	2 (5%)	40
Peritoneal dialysis	8 (61.5%)	4 (30.8%)	1 (7.7%)	13
Intravenous fluids containing sodium	27 (84.4%)	3 (9.4%)	2 (6.2%)	32
Supportive only	54 (77.1%)	8 (11.4%)	8 (11.4%)	70
Forced diuresis	8			8
Mannitol	5	1	1	7
Unspecified	7	10	1	18
Total	143	30	15	188

*This group includes cases in which the presence or absence of sequelae may not have been specified.
**Percentage given a specific therapy.
Source. Reprinted from El-Mallakh 1986a. Used with permission.

Postmortem brain lithium levels have been reported in some cases (Table 3–5). However, the delay between initial presentation, death, and obtaining the brain following death makes interpretation of the data quite difficult.

Optimal treatment for acute toxicity is dictated by the clinical course and the serum lithium levels. In severe cases, hemodialysis is the treatment of choice (El-Mallakh 1986a). Limited reports,

Table 3–5. Postmortem lithium levels in the serum and areas of the human brain

Organ[a]	Patient (age & sex)											
	30 M	71 F	47 F	43 F						56 F	71	41 F
Serum (mEq/L)	1.3		1.93	0.5	0.25	0.35						0.3
Cerebrum, grey				0.72	0.15	0.24					1.2	
Cerebrum, white				0.85	0.18	0.34					1.6	0.44
Cerebrum, unspecified	0.0	1.4	1.41				17.0	2.9	13.5	1.13		0.75
Cerebellum, grey				0.35				3.5				6.5 (2.1)[b]
Cerebellum, unspecified				0.51						0.6		
Pons					0.35	0.65	0.7	1.9				
Midbrain							89.6	1.9	12.2			
Amygdala												
Hippocampus							9.7	6.2	12.5			0.36
Cerebrospinal fluid	1.0											0.89

[a] All values are in mEq/kg wet weight unless otherwise specified.
[b] This value is in mEq/kg dry weight.
Source. Reprinted from El-Mallakh 1986a. Used with permission.

mainly from Europe, have shown adequate results with peritoneal dialysis (El-Mallakh 1986a). Patients with less severe cases are usually supported until lithium is eliminated by the kidneys. The use of sodium to provide an "internal dialysis," that is, to accelerate lithium efflux from cells (El-Mallakh 1984), has not been adequately stressed in the literature. Sodium is important because the major route of efflux of intracellular lithium is via the sodium–lithium counterexchange system (El-Mallakh 1983b, 1990b; Pandey et al. 1978). Note that although this activity reduces the toxic intracellular lithium, it may actually increase serum lithium levels. This store of intracellular lithium is also responsible for lithium level rebound after a session of hemodialysis (i.e., the increase in serum lithium levels seen within the first few hours after hemodialysis; see Escobar and Skoutakis 1979).

CNS manifestations can also occur as chronic side effects. In some patients, tremor and deep tendon reflex changes may be persistent side effects. At therapeutic levels, lithium may also cause a subjective and objective decrease in cognitive functioning (Ananth et al. 1987; Glue et al. 1987). Although many studies are flawed by poor methodology or the effects of the affective illness itself (El-Mallakh 1990a), healthy volunteers on chronic therapeutic levels of lithium exhibited a discrete reduction in the ability to perform associative mental tasks (Glue et al. 1987).

Long-term therapeutic lithium therapy has also been shown to produce a nonspecific slowing of the EEG activity (Itil and Akpinar 1971). Most often, there is an increase in theta and delta activity, with a simultaneous decrease in alpha waves. Because of this pattern, lithium was classified as a neuroleptic by Fink (1969). These EEG changes appear as a function of lithium dosage and the chronicity of therapy (G. Johnson 1969; Mayfield and Brown 1966; Platman and Fieve 1969; Small et al. 1971b). Thus, one 750-mg dose of lithium does not produce any EEG change, whereas a dose of 1,000–2,500 mg daily over several days will cause changes in 70% of patients (G. Johnson et al. 1970). Similarly, several investigators have documented the slowing of peripheral nerve conduction velocities that correlated with lithium level and chronicity of administration (Chang et al. 1990; Girke et al. 1975; Manocha et al. 1984).

ACUTE AND CHRONIC CARDIOTOXICITY

Specific cardiac manifestations of acute lithium toxicity are rare. Most reports of cardiovascular collapse (Tilkian et al. 1976a, 1976b) describe terminal events in patients who had severe, late-stage neurotoxicity (coma and seizures). However, several cases describing sinoatrial nodal blockade (Eliasen and Andersen 1975; Roose et al. 1979b; Tobin et al. 1974; Wellens et al. 1975; Wilson et al. 1976), frequently with dizziness, syncope, or exertional dyspnea, at therapeutic lithium levels, are clearly describing lithium cardiotoxicity. Other noted lithium cardiotoxic effects are an increased ventricular irritability with increased frequency of premature ventricular beats (Tangedahl and Gau 1972; Tilkian et al. 1976a, 1976b) and decreased cardiac condition with atrioventricular blockade, intraventricular conduction delays, and prolongation of the A–T interval (Jacob and Hope 1979; Jaffe 1977; Mateer and Clark 1982; Mitchell and MacKenzie 1982; Roose et al. 1979a; Tilkian et al. 1976b). All of these changes have been reported to occur at both therapeutic and toxic lithium level ranges.

These lithium-induced conduction abnormalities resemble the antiarrhythmic effects of verapamil and diltiazem (Mauritson et al. 1982; McGoon et al. 1982; Sung et al. 1980). These primary cardiovascular agents delay conduction by interfering with calcium transport across myocardial cell membranes (Mauritson et al. 1982; McGoon et al. 1982; Sung et al. 1980). Likewise, lithium may act as a calcium entry inhibitor (El-Mallakh 1983b). The mechanism of calcium entry blockade is probably different, and lithium is probably less effective at blocking calcium entry in myocardial tissues than the calcium channel blockers (see Chapter 6). Nonetheless, in the myocardium, the combined calcium entry blocking action of lithium and the calcium channel blockers is probably additive, and acute cardiotoxicity with combined therapy has been reported (Dubovsky et al. 1987).

More chronic, less clinically significant cardiac response to lithium therapy involves reversible, asymptomatic electrocardiographic changes. Changes are limited to T wave flattening, depression, and inversion and resemble changes seen with hypokalemia. Lithium produces a relative intracellular hypokalemia (El-Mallakh 1983b;

Tilkian et al. 1976b). Various authors have placed the incidence of these changes at anywhere between 20% and 100% of patients receiving lithium (Demers and Heninger 1971; Mitchell and Mac-Kenzie 1982; Schou 1963b; Tilkian et al. 1976b). In some reports of cardiac pathology in patients receiving lithium, the etiological role of lithium is questionable. Two complicated cases of fatal myocarditis in patients receiving lithium have attracted significant attention (Swedberg and Winblad 1974; Tseng 1971). One patient had hypothyroidism, latent syphilis, and an undiagnosed generalized skin lesion (Tseng 1971); the other also suffered from hypothyroidism and preexisting cardiac failure (Swedberg and Winblad 1974). Nonetheless, there are reasons to suspect that lithium may play a role in producing myocarditis (Tilkian et al. 1976b). As stated earlier, lithium produces a relative intracellular hypokalemia (El-Mallakh 1983b; Tilkian et al. 1976b), and severe potassium depletion, and hypokalemia may produce a myocarditis in both animals and humans (Ananth et al. 1987; Harrison et al. 1972; Rodriguez et al. 1950). Obviously, the rarity of this complication suggests that it is primarily of theoretical concern. Reports of myocardial infarctions in patients receiving lithium (Baldessarini and Stephens 1970; Schwartz and Lopez-Toca 1982; Warick 1979) probably represent a coexistence of separate and unrelated conditions. Lithium may actually be protective; in the trace amounts found in mineral-laden (hard) water, lithium was associated with a decreased incidence of both sudden death and atherosclerotic heart disease (Anderson et al. 1969; Voors 1970).

Finally, despite the recognized arrhythmogenic effects of phenothiazines (Fowler et al. 1976) and the high frequency with which they are coadministered with lithium, there are very few reported combined cardiotoxic manifestations (Baastrup et al. 1976; Goldney and Spence 1986; Salama 1987). These findings suggest that the cardiotoxic mechanisms of lithium and phenothiazines, or neuroleptics in general, may not be additive.

RENAL TOXICITY

The most frequent renal side effects of lithium treatment are polyuria and polydipsia (Lyskowski et al. 1982; Reisberg and Gershon 1979). Lithium produces an initial diuresis in as many as

50% of patients. This result decreases to approximately 25% of patients on long-term treatment (Lyskowski et al. 1982; Reisberg and Gershon 1979). There are two causes for lithium-induced polyuria. The first cause (a very mild and reversible, dose-related polyuria) is related to the large hydration radius of the lithium ion (Schou 1957); that is, when lithium is excreted by the kidney, a large amount of water molecules must accompany it. The second, and a more severe, cause (vasopressin-unresponsive, but reversible, impaired concentrating ability) is nephrogenic diabetes insipidus (NDI) (Forrest et al. 1974). NDI appears to result from lithium's interference with vasopressin-activated cyclic adenosine monophosphate (cAMP) (Dousa and Hechter 1970; Forrest et al. 1974). Lithium decreases the kidney's sensitivity to both endogenously produced and exogenously administered vasopressin (Forrest et al. 1974). This effect is not significant enough to reverse fluid retention in the syndrome of inappropriate secretion of antidiuretic hormones (Forrest et al. 1978). Generally, polyuria is not considered to be an omen of worsening renal functions (Lippmann 1982), but this view is disputed (H. E. Hansen et al. 1979; Santella et al. 1988). It is certain, however, that severe polyuria may reduce patient compliance and may also pose a greater potential for lithium toxicity if oral fluid intake is insufficient (El-Mallakh 1986a; Thomsen and Olesen 1978). Consequently, several schemes to reduce polyuria have been attempted.

Because urinary lithium excretion removes a large amount of body water, methods of retaining lithium would decrease polyuria. Capitalizing on the differential handling of sodium and lithium by the kidney, several researchers have recommended thiazide diuretics (Battle et al. 1985; Forrest et al. 1974; Himmelhoch et al. 1977a, 1977b; Lippmann et al. 1981; Poust et al. 1976). Both sodium and lithium are readily reabsorbed by the proximal tubule, but at normal sodium levels, lithium is not reabsorbed by the distal nephron (Lippmann et al. 1981). Thiazide diuretics cause sodium wasting by preventing sodium reabsorption in the distal tubule, thus increasing both sodium and lithium retention by the proximal tubule. The decreased lithium clearance reduces the water loss and ameliorates the polyuria (Lippmann et al. 1981). As more lithium is retained by the kidney, significant reductions in lithium doses are usually needed (Himmelhoch et al. 1977a, 1977b;

Lippmann et al. 1981). If distal tubule diuretics are used, maintaining normal sodium levels becomes extremely important. Because the distal tubule will reabsorb lithium in hyponatremic settings (Boer et al. 1987), sudden sodium loss may cause serum lithium levels to rise. Nonetheless, various studies have shown that with appropriate caution, lithium and diuretics can be coadministered (Battle et al. 1985; Himmelhoch et al. 1977a, 1977b; Lippmann et al. 1981; Poust et al. 1976). Still, the frequent presentation of acute lithium toxicity soon after the initiation of diuretic therapy (El-Mallakh 1986a; Nurnberger 1985) prevents the widespread use of diuretics.

It is noteworthy that diuretics reduce water loss by reducing lithium loss but do not address the cAMP-vasopressin mechanism directly. Vasopressin response has not been investigated in either animal or human thiazide-treated lithium polyuria.

In rare cases, severe polyuria may persist after lithium treatment has been discontinued (Brooks and Lessin 1983; Rabin et al. 1979). Although thiazide diuretics may be useful in such cases (E. Z. Rabin et al. 1979), the novel use of carbamazepine to treat both the manic behavior and NDI has been successful in at least one case (Brooks and Lessin 1983).

Glomerular function may also be affected by chronic lithium treatment. Researchers have suggested that there may be a slight decrease in glomerular filtration over time, which, for the majority of patients, appears to be clinically unimportant but nonetheless warrants the monitoring of serum creatinine (Decina et al. 1983; Jorkasky et al. 1985; Santella et al. 1988).

Much more serious have been the reports of histologically documented nephropathies (Alexander and Martia 1981; Baer and Paul 1985; Burrows et al. 1978; Depner 1982; H. E. Hansen et al. 1979; Hestbech and Aurell 1979; Lippmann 1982; Richman et al. 1980; Santella et al. 1988). In 1977, Hestbech et al. reported 14 patients who had suffered an episode of acute lithium toxicity or had lithium-induced NDI. The researchers described interstitial fibrosis, tubular atrophy, and sclerotic glomeruli on biopsy and autopsy specimens (Hestbech et al. 1977). Other similar reports were published through the late 1970s and early 1980s (Baer and Paul 1985; Burrows et al. 1978; H. E. Hansen et al. 1979; Lippmann 1982). However, most of these reports did not use appropriate controls. When the renal function of lithium-treated patients was compared with patients with affective illness on psychotropic medications other than lithium, no significant differences were noted (Hullin et al. 1979). Likewise, when renal biopsy specimens were compared among normal kidney donors, affective disorder patients on lithium, and affective disorder patients before lithium was initiated, it was noted that kidney abnormalities were more prevalent among the affective disorder patients and that these changes were independent of their exposure to lithium (Kincaid-Smith et al. 1979). The presence of similar lesions in the appropriate control group raises valid questions as to the significance of the earlier reports.

Reports of lithium-related nephrotic syndrome have continued to appear (Alexander and Martia 1981; Baer and Paul 1985; Depner 1982; Richman et al. 1980; Santella et al. 1988), and, to date, 11 have been described (Santella et al. 1988). These patients have either minimal change, tubulointerstitial disease, or glomerulosclerosis (Santella et al. 1988). The variable histology and the small number of cases suggest concurrent separate diseases. However, the fact that in most cases the nephrosis either improved or remitted completely when lithium was discontinued and that lithium rechallenge produced a recurrence in three patients (Santella et al. 1988) suggests a cause-effect relationship or at least a permissive role of lithium.

Finally, acute severe lithium toxicity has been reported to produce oliguric renal failure (Dias and Hochen 1972; Lavender et al. 1973). If the patient survives the acute toxic episode, renal function returns to normal (Lavender et al. 1973). Notably, the picture in these patients is often complicated with preexisting anorexia, diarrhea, and dehydration, and the question of a prerenal cause for the renal shutdown (other than lithium) has never been adequately addressed. Histological abnormalities in this group are not significantly different from those in patients who never experience toxic episodes (Dias and Hochen 1972; H. E. Hansen et al. 1979; Hestbech et al. 1977; Lavender et al. 1973).

ENDOCRINE SIDE EFFECTS

Lithium affects a variety of endocrine systems. As mentioned in the renal section, lithium inhibits the vasopressin activation of adenyl cyclase and subsequent cAMP-mediated events. Lithium also affects thyroid, parathyroid, and glucose metabolism.

Thyroid

Lithium decreases the sensitivity of the thyroid gland to the thyroid-stimulating hormone (TSH) and inhibits both TSH-induced thyroxine release and colloid droplet formation (Emerson et al. 1973). As with NDI, lithium appears to interfere with the TSH second messenger, cAMP (Singer and Rotenberg 1973). This lithium-induced resistance to TSH causes an increase in plasma levels of TSH in 10%–30% of patients receiving lithium (Emerson et al. 1973; Lindstedt et al. 1977; Mannisto 1980; Stern and Lydiard 1987; Transbol et al. 1978). In most cases, this increase is enough to maintain a euthyroid state, but 3%–5% of patients will go on to develop a euthyroid goiter (Schou et al. 1968; Shopsin 1970; Stern and Lydiard 1987), and perhaps another 3%–5% may become hypothyroid (Mannisto 1980; Shopsin 1970; Stern and Lydiard 1987). Lithium has been advocated for the treatment of hyperthyroidism but is rarely used clinically (Temple et al. 1972). Rare instances of lithium-associated exophthalmos and hyperthyroidism remain unexplained (P. L. Rabin and Evans 1981; Segal et al. 1973). Attempts to implicate antithyroid antibodies in the pathogenesis of these various thyroid abnormalities have not provided consistent results (Calabrese et al. 1985; Lazarus et al. 1986; Leroy et al. 1988).

Parathyroid and Calcium Metabolism

Lithium has been reported to produce a mild increase in free calcium as well as a clinical hypercalcemia (Cervi-Skinner 1977; Feinberg et al. 1979; Mallette and Eichhort 1986; McIntosh et al. 1987), but these findings are disputed (Aronoff et al. 1971; Spiegel et al. 1984). Other researchers have documented increased levels of parathyroid hormone (PTH) along with increased calcium (Christiansen et al. 1980; Mallette and Eichhort 1986; McIntosh et al. 1987; Nielsen et al. 1977). Furthermore, lithium has been found to stimulate the direct release of PTH in vitro from bovine (E. M. Brown 1981) and human (Birnbaum et al. 1988) parathyroid tissue at levels comparable to those produced by low calcium. The mechanism of this is unclear but may be related to lithium's ability to indirectly displace active free intracellular calcium (El-Mallakh 1983b). Aside from the apparent accidental coexistence of parathyroid adenomas (McIntosh et al. 1987), the effects of lithium on calcium and PTH do not appear to be clinically significant.

Glucose Metabolism

Lithium has an antidiabetic effect in both humans (Saran 1982; van der Velde and Gordon 1969; Weiss 1924) and animals (Mannisto and Koivisto 1972). Lithium promotes the direct uptake of the glucose derivative 3-O-methyl glucose by body tissues in vitro (Kohn and Clausen 1972) and increases glycogen storage in various tissues (Plenge et al. 1970). This insulin-like effect increases plasma glucagon and decreases liver glycogen stores (Mellerup et al. 1970). Some of lithium's effect may be mediated by its ability to interrupt the metabolism of glucagon-mediated cAMP (El-Mallakh 1983b, 1986b). Clinically, this antidiabetic effect has two major implications: 1) As previously stated, in some diabetic patients, readjustment of the insulin or hypoglycemic agent dose may be required. 2) In nearly 30% of nondiabetic patients receiving lithium, this insulin-like effect may cause a nonfluid weight gain (Dempsey et al. 1976; Kerry et al. 1979).

TERATOGENICITY

Lithium given during the critical first trimester of pregnancy is a recognized teratogen. Through data gathered by the International Register of Lithium Babies, it was found that 11% of babies born to mothers taking lithium and reported to the register were born with congenital abnormalities (compared with 3% in the general population) (Weinstein 1980). Of the total malformations, 72% were cardiovascular abnormalities (compared with 12.5% in the general population) (Weinstein 1980). Ebstein's anomaly of the tricuspid valve has been noted to be the most frequent in the register data (33.3% versus 1.2% in the general population) and by other researchers (Nora et al. 1974; Weinstein 1980). A Swedish cohort study found an incidence of 7% of congenital heart defects among offspring of bipolar women on lithium, compared with 1% in offspring of bipolar women not on lithium (Kallen and Tandberg 1983). This study, which has superior methodology over the register data, did not document a high incidence of Ebstein's anomaly (Kallen and Tandberg 1983).

There are conflicting data regarding lithium-induced chromosomal abnormalities (Garson et al. 1981; Torre and Krompotic 1976). However, because lithium inhibits DNA polymerase activity (Lazarus and Kitron 1974), genetic abnormalities may be quite likely. Animals receiving more than 10 times the therapeutic human dose develop a host of developmental abnormalities (Szabo 1969; Wright et al. 1970).

MISCELLANEOUS EFFECTS

Lithium has been reported to have various effects on skin, including psoriasis, dermatitis, and alopecia (Labelle and Lapierre 1991; Reisberg and Gershon 1979; Sarantidis and Waters 1983; Shukla and Mukherjee 1984; Silvestri et al. 1988). Worsening of the complexion and acne are particularly important determinants of poor compliance in adolescents.

Effects on respiratory function have also been reported. Despite a report of two cases of coincidental improvement of asthma at therapeutic lithium dosages (Nasr and Atkins 1977), lithium has been shown to decrease respiratory compensation in the face of increased inspiratory resistance (Weiner et al. 1983). Although these findings are not mutually exclusive, they suggest differing levels of concern. Lithium therapy should be reevaluated in the clinical setting of deteriorating respiratory status.

SUMMARY

Although lithium's narrow therapeutic index makes toxicity a constant concern, the toxic consequences of lithium therapy and overdosage may be valuable clues to understanding the mechanisms of lithium action. Among the key points are the widespread hormonal disruption; the predilection of the nervous system to toxicity, with relative sparing of other electrically active tissue such as the heart and skeletal muscle; and the occasionally opposite clinical effects of therapeutic lithium levels (e.g., anticonvulsant and antimanic properties) and toxic lithium levels (convulsant and manicogenic).

Section II

Mechanisms of Lithium Action

Chapter 4

Lithium and First Messengers

N early all of the major early efforts to understand the mechanism of action of lithium focused on neurotransmitters and their receptors—collectively referred to as *first messengers*. These efforts were direct consequences of various attempts to understand bipolar illness itself. Thus, models of lithium action always attempted to support hypotheses of bipolar pathogenesis.

The experimental data have been insufficient to support any one model of lithium action on first messengers to the exclusion of others. More recently, this approach has been largely abandoned in favor of more instructive second-messenger studies (see Chapter 5). In this chapter, I briefly review some of the highlights of these studies.

BIOGENIC AMINES

The biogenic amine hypotheses for mood disorders grew out of the catecholamine hypothesis, originally formulated in the mid-1960s (Bunney and Davis 1965; Prange 1964; Schildkraut 1965). These hypotheses were constructed, and later modified and expanded, on the basis of pharmacological actions of certain drugs. Specifically, resperine, which depletes central nervous system (CNS) catecholamines, may induce depression. Monoamine oxidase–inhibiting agents, which increase CNS amines, and tricyclic antidepressants, which increase the postsynaptic availability of amines by blocking reuptake, have antidepressant properties. These early hypotheses did not distinguish unipolar and bipolar depression. The theories proposed that all biological depressions resulted from brain amine deficiency and that mania resulted from excesses of these compounds. Thus, lithium was proposed to affect these neurotransmitters by normalizing their levels.

Although catecholamine neuron systems constitute < 1% of the total mammalian neuron population, they are, nonetheless, widely distributed throughout the brain. Norepinephrine is a neuromodulator that innervates the entire CNS from two nuclei located in the brain stem (Moore 1982). Neocortical norepinephrine neurons originate in the locus coeruleus, a pigmented nucleus also containing neuromelanin (Moore 1982). Additional norepinephrine neurons originate from the lateral and dorsal medullary reticular formations, which innervate predominantly lower brain structures. Neurons from these nuclei are distinctive in being highly collateralized, with each one synapting with hundreds or thousands of cortical neurons. Furthermore, the morphology of these synapses is unusual in that typical synaptic complexes are infrequent. Rather, norepinephrine neocortical terminals terminate in such a way as to distribute their effects beyond the immediate terminal junction (Moore 1982). Consequently, although specific functions of the noradrenergic system remain unknown, it is reasonable to assume that they are involved in the modulation of the potency of other neurotransmitter systems (Moore 1982).

As such, norepinephrine can be viewed as a good candidate for the extensive symptomatic involvement observed in mood disorders. The hypothesis that norepinephrine deficiency was involved in the pathogenesis of depression, while its excess produced mania, was further supported by studies that found that norepinephrine metabolites were decreased in bipolar depression (Bond et al. 1972; Greenspan et al. 1970b; Jones et al. 1973; Maas 1975; Strom-Olsen and Weil-Malherebe 1958) and unipolar depression (Maas 1975; Schildkraut et al. 1978; C. M. Shaw et al. 1973) and elevated in hypomania and mania (Bond et al. 1972; Greenspan et al. 1970b; Jones et al. 1973; Maas 1975; Strom-Olsen and Weil-Malherebe 1958).

Dopamine is another catecholamine that has an extensive limbic and striatal distribution. Biochemically, dopamine is a precursor to norepinephrine. Physiologically, dopamine shares some of the unique characteristics of norepinephrine noted above (Moore 1982). Neuroleptics, by virtue of their dopamine-blocking ability, have well-documented antimanic properties (Chouinard and Steiner 1986; Goodwin and Zis 1979), whereas various classes of dopamine-agonist agents can precipitate manic states in bipolar patients (Gerner et al. 1976; Murphy et al. 1971a; Silverstone 1984). A role for dopamine in depression has not been generally advocated, but dopamine is believed to play a role in the more severe manifestations of bipolar psychosis (Goodwin and Jamison 1990).

Serotonin is an indolamine synthesized from tryptophan. It, too, is a neuromodulator, originating in the brain stem raphe nucleus and projecting throughout the brain. It appears to have a general moderating or inhibitory effect, and its depletion is associated with the disinhibition of behavior. Several lines of evidence, including cerebrospinal fluid (CSF) levels of the serotonin metabolite 5-hydroxyindoleacetic acid (5-HIAA) (Åsberg et al. 1976; Coppen et al. 1972; Goodwin and Jamison 1990; van Praag et al. 1973) and platelet serotonin levels (Coppen et al. 1978; Tuomisto and Tukiainen 1976), suggest that serotonin activity is decreased in both mania and depression. This evidence has led to the generally accepted serotonin-permissive hypothesis of mood disorders, which proposes that the absence of the moderating action of serotonin allows for the extreme swings of bipolar illness (Goodwin and Jamison 1990).

The literature discussing the relative merits and shortfalls of any of these hypotheses is extensive and beyond the scope of this discussion. Certainly none of the amine hypotheses is exclusive of the others. However, the effects of lithium treatment on the various amines, and its mechanism of action within the framework of these first-messenger hypotheses, are quite unclear.

Lithium and Biogenic Amines

There are no consistent effects of lithium on brain amine turnover, synthesis, or release (Bliss and Ailion 1970; Corrodi et al. 1969; Friedman and Gershon 1973; Greenspan et al. 1970a; Ho et al. 1970; Knapp and Mandell 1973; L. H. Price et al. 1990; Schildkraut 1973), and most studies find no change in levels of biogenic amines and their metabolites in animals chronically treated with lithium (Bliss and Ailion 1970; Corrodi et al. 1969; Greenspan et al. 1970a; Ho et al. 1970). Animal data are further confused by the lack of standardized methods. Nearly all studies have a different duration of treatment, route and dosage of lithium administration, and methods of estimating amine turnover.

Human studies are nearly as fruitless. Lithium has been reported to decrease (Greenspan et al. 1970b; Messiha et al. 1970), increase (Mendels 1971; L. H. Price et al. 1990; Wilk et al. 1972), or not change (Bowers et al. 1969; Haskovec and Rysanek 1969; L. H. Price et al. 1990) CSF, blood and urinary levels of biogenic amines and their metabolites. These findings are perhaps not too surprising because lithium does not appear to interact directly with any of these receptors or neurotransmitters. That is, first-messenger changes consequent to lithium treatment are expected to be downstream effects that could be variably altered by the original illness, environmental effects, and treatment.

One consistently reproduced effect of chronic lithium treatment has been its ability to block haloperidol-induced behavioral supersensitivity to the dopamine-agonist apomorphine (Potter 1993). This ability has been interpreted as an attenuation of haloperidol-induced receptor supersensitivity (Gallager et al. 1978; Pert et al. 1978). Clinically, this attenuation may be seen as a partial protection from the development of tardive dyskinesia in patients receiving both lithium and neuroleptic agents (see Chapter 3) (Mukherjee et al. 1986; Waddington and Youssef 1988). Blocking receptor supersensitivity may be a more general effect of lithium. For example, some authors report that lithium can prevent muscarinic receptor supersensitivity (see below).

ACETYLCHOLINE

Acetylcholine is a widely distributed neurotransmitter in the brain that arises mainly from the large (> 30 μm) hyperchromic neurons of the basal forebrain, usually referred to as the *nucleus basalas of Meynert* (El-Mallakh et al. 1991; Ezrin-Waters and Resch 1986). Acetylcholine plays a significant role in learning, memory, and arousal (Richardson and DeLong 1988), and deficiency has been implicated in a wide variety of dementing illnesses (Cummings and Benson 1987).

In the peripheral nervous system, acetylcholine is the major parasympathetic neurotransmitter, balanced by sympathetic (norepinephrine and epinephrine) activity. Janowsky et al. (1972) proposed that a similar acetylcholine–norepinephrine balance in the CNS may underlie mood disorders; specifically, a relative increase of central acetylcholine could produce depression, whereas a relative decrease may produce mania. In support of this hypothesis, several groups have reported that physostigmine (a cholinesterase inhibitor that prevents the hydrolysis of acetylcholine and therefore extends its activity) can transiently reverse manic symptoms (K. L. Davis et al. 1978; Janowsky et al. 1973; Modestin et al. 1973) or precipitate depressive symptoms in euthymic, lithium-treated bipolar patients (Oppenheim et al. 1979).

Lithium and Acetylcholine

Lithium apparently interferes with choline transport. Thus, in lithium-treated patients, intraerythrocyte choline may be 10 times more concentrated than plasma choline, which does not change (Goodnick and Shapiro 1993; C. S. Tang and Miller 1993). Furthermore, the extent of intraerythrocyte choline rise appears to be related to clinical response (Goodnick and Shapiro, 1993). However, because choline transport is coupled to norepinephrine, this effect may be secondary to lithium-induced alterations in norepinephrine transport (see Chapter 6) (Goodnick and Shapiro 1993). The CNS consequences of elevated intracellular choline are unclear (Goodnick and Shapiro 1993; C. S. Tang and Miller 1993), and they probably do not persist with long-term treatment (C. S. Tang and Miller 1993).

More interestingly, chronic lithium treatment has been reported by some (Ellis and Lenox 1990; Levy et al. 1983), although not all (Lerer and Stanley 1985), to prevent acetylcholine receptor supersensitivity. Lithium does so without altering the acetylcholine receptor binding (Ellis and Lenox 1990; Lerer and Stanley 1985; Levy et al. 1983; Maggi and Enna 1982; Tollefson and Senogles 1982). This may be an important observation because acetylcholine receptor supersensitivity is believed to play a pathogenic role in mood disorders (Dilsaver 1984, 1986).

As noted above, the lithium-induced prevention of antagonist-mediated acetylcholine- and dopamine-receptor supersensitivity may be a reflection of a more general consequence of lithium treatment. This sensitivity may not be directly related to first messengers but is more likely related to an alteration in second-messenger function (see Chapter 5) or nonselective decreased synaptic neurotransmitter release (see Chapter 6).

GAMMA-AMINOBUTYRIC ACID

Gamma-aminobutyric acid (GABA) is the major inhibitory amino acid neurotransmitter in the CNS. Unlike the substances discussed previously, GABA acts more like a true neurotransmitter than a neuromodulator. Both GABA receptor subtypes produce immediate and relatively short-term inhibition of postsynaptic neural excitation (Sivilotti and Nistri 1991). $GABA_A$ increases chloride conductance (i.e., chloride influx), thereby hyperpolarizing the neuron by increasing the relative intracellular negative charge (Sivilotti and Nistri 1991). $GABA_B$ increases potassium conductance (i.e., potassium influx), thereby hyperpolarizing the neuron by moving the transmembrane potential closer to the potassium potential (see Chapter 6) (Sivilotti and Nistri 1991). Unlike the amines and acetylcholine, GABAergic neurons are not limited to or originating at a few nuclei but are much more diffusely distributed throughout the brain. GABA is involved in the modulation of nearly all CNS activity, so it is not surprising that GABA has been implicated in the pathophysiology of mania (Goodwin and Jamison 1990; Motohashi 1993).

The proposal that a GABA deficiency may produce both mania and depression is based on mechanisms of various classes of thymoleptics. Mood stabilizers effective in bipolar illness, particularly valproate and carbamazepine and perhaps lithium as well, appear to enhance GABA transmission (Goodwin and Jamison 1990; Motohashi 1993). Furthermore, antidepressant drugs may potentiate GABA via $GABA_B$ receptors (Goodwin and Jamison 1990), and the benzodiazepine alprazolam appears to have antidepressant properties (at least in short-term treatment) (Feighner et al. 1983; Rickels et al. 1985).

Lithium and GABA

Lithium treatment and remission are associated with an increase in both plasma and CSF GABA levels (Berrettini et al. 1983;

Motohashi 1993), perhaps to levels even higher than in normal control subjects (Perry and Sherman 1984). This finding was predicted by Berl and Clarke in 1975 because of lithium's ability to reduce the glial uptake of glutamate and GABA. These researchers argued that if the neurotransmitters are not taken up and inactivated, then they would eventually spill over into the CSF (Berl and Clarke 1975). However, in animal studies, GABA synthesis does not change in a reliable fashion, and turnover is decreased (Motohashi 1993; Berl and Clarke 1975), whereas $GABA_B$ receptors are upregulated (Motohashi et al. 1989).

NEUROPEPTIDES AND FATTY ACIDS

In animals, lithium increases the synthesis and levels of neuropeptide Y, SP, somatostatin, neurokinin A, calcitonin gene–related peptide, and neurotensin (Mathé et al. 1993). Unfortunately, the current poor level of understanding of the physiological actions of these peptides precludes any conclusions.

Similarly, fatty acids and prostaglandins have been implicated in mood disorders (Hibbeln et al. 1989; Horrobin 1990), and lithium can disrupt various aspects of fat metabolism (Harvey et al. 1993). Lithium's effects on fatty acids are believed to modify neuronal function by modifying second messengers (Harvey et al. 1993) or membrane fluidity (N. E. Joseph et al. 1987). Unfortunately, the low level of experimental activity in this area, coupled with attempts to understand lithium mechanisms within the framework of a complex and poorly understood system, make conclusions difficult to reach. (It should be noted that the decision to not explore these fields in detail in this book does not reflect a belief that this work is unimportant. On the contrary, work with neuropeptides and fatty acid metabolism will probably represent a major force in future lithium research.)

SUMMARY

Bipolar illness affects all aspects of brain function. The sensory, motor, cognitive, emotional, autonomic, and endocrine systems may all be dysfunctional in the course of mania, bipolar depression, or both. All of these aspects respond to treatment with lithium. It is thus likely that lithium modifies the action of a widely distributed substance or process. The neurotransmitter GABA and the neuromodulators norepinephrine, dopamine, serotonin, and acetylcholine all modulate a wide array of brain functions, vary with various somatic treatments of mania or depression, and have been implicated in the pathophysiology of bipolar illness. However, the evidence that the prophylactic and therapeutic actions of lithium are mediated via these first messengers is not particularly impressive.

Lithium appears to alter some aspect of function for each neuromodulator and neurotransmitter discussed. However, these changes are not readily reproducible and occur despite a lack of direct interaction between lithium and the first messengers. It appears likely that first-messenger changes are secondary to the well-documented effects on second-messenger systems (see Chapter 5) and cellular ionic regulation (see Chapter 6). For example, the observed prevention of dopamine and acetylcholine receptor supersensitivity could be a result of nonspecific interference with neurotransmitter release (Chapter 6). Similarly, changes in sodium-dependent choline and GABA transport could be caused by alterations of relative sodium gradients or a modification of sodium-lithium countertransport systems (Chapter 6).

Although it is important to investigate the consequences of lithium therapy on first messengers, experimental experience has shown that a greater understanding of lithium mechanisms can be achieved by investigating second-messenger and nonspecific ionic flux effects.

Chapter 5

Observations on Second-Messenger Systems

Most neurotransmitters and neuromodulators will exert two major actions at a postsynaptic cell—an immediate effect and a delayed effect. The immediate neurotransmitter effect is mediated by plasma membrane ion channels and results in a potentiation (e.g., glutamate) or attenuation (e.g., gamma-aminobutyric acid [GABA]) of a postsynaptic action potential. The delayed neuromodulator effect is mediated by second messengers and may be evident for seconds to minutes after neurotransmitter-receptor interaction. Although the immediate effect is what ultimately results in measurable neuronal activity, the delayed, second-messenger–mediated action of neurotransmitters is now becoming recognized as a major force in the regulation and function of neurons. Two of the best studied neuronal second-messenger systems are the adenylate cyclase system and the phosphatidylinositol/diacylglycerol (PI/DAG) system (Figure 5–1). Lithium has been found to affect the second-message signal of a wide variety of both stimulatory and inhibitory neurotransmitters, always in the direction of reducing signal intensity.

The general sequence of receptor-activated intracellular events is represented in Figure 5–1 (Baraban et al. 1989; Berridge 1984; Gilman 1987). Interaction of a neurotransmitter or agonist with the cellular-membrane receptor, in the presence of magnesium and guanosine triphosphate (GTP), results in the activation of a membrane G protein (so-called because of its dependence on GTP). The activated G protein complex will interact with adenylate cyclase or phospholipase C to produce the respective second messenger (Figure 5–1).

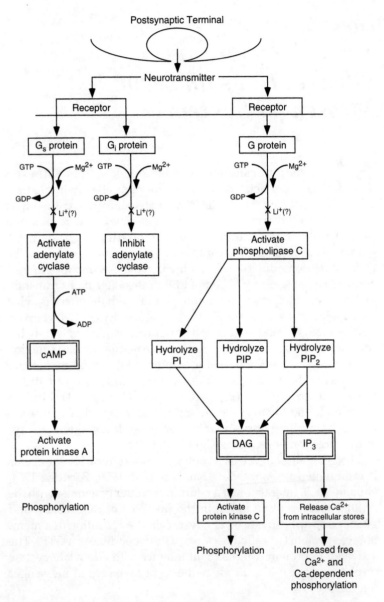

Figure 5–1.   The cAMP and PI/DAG second-messenger systems.

All G proteins share the same general organization (Figure 5–2). Inactive G proteins are composed of three subunits (α, β, δ). In response to agonist receptor activation, and in the presence of magnesium, GTP binds to the α subunit—displacing the $\beta\delta$ subunit

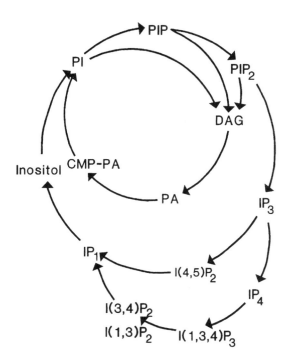

Figure 5–2. A greatly simplified phosphoinositide cycle. Only DAG and IP$_3$ have recognized second-messenger functions, but other intermediates may also be biologically active. Abbreviations: CMP-PA = cytidine monophosphorylaphosphatidate; DAG=diacylglycerol; IP$_1$ = any of three forms, inositol 4-monophosphate, inositol 1-monophosphate, or inositol 3-monophosphate; I(4,5) P$_2$ = inositol 1,4-bisphosphate; I(1,3)P$_2$ = inositol 1,3-bisphosphate; I(3,4) P$_2$ = inositol 3,4-bisphosphate; IP$_3$ = inositol 1,4,5-triphosphate; I(1,3,4) P$_3$ = inositol 1,3,4 triphosphate; IP$_4$ = inositol 1,3,4,5-tetrakisphosphate; PA = phosphatidic acid; PI = phosphatidylinositol; PIP = phosphatidylinositol 4-monophosphate; PIP$_2$ = phosphatidylinositol 4,5-bisphosphate.

complex and freeing the α subunit from the agonist-receptor complex (Figure 5–2). It is the free α subunit that interacts with either adenylate cyclase or phospholipase C. The α subunit also possesses magnesium-dependent GTPase activity and will dephosphorylate GTP to guanosine diphosphate (GDP), thereby allowing for reassociation with βδ and the termination of G protein activation (Figure 5–2) (Baraban et al. 1989; Gilman 1987).

Magnesium is important in this sequence of events. G proteins possess at least two magnesium sites. A high-affinity (nM range) site is required for the hydrolysis of GTP, whereas a low-affinity site (mM range) is required for the βδ subunit complex-GTP exchange (Brandt and Ross 1986; Gilman 1987; Higashijima et al. 1987). Neurotransmitters stimulate G protein-GTP coupling, in part, by changing the magnesium requirement for the low-affinity site to the μM range (Brandt and Ross 1986; Iyengar and Birnbaumer 1982). Normal total intracellular magnesium concentrations measured by atomic absorption spectrophotometry in erythrocytes are 2–2.5 mM (Frazer et al. 1972; Paolisso et al. 1988; Ramsey et al. 1979a; Sjögren et al. 1988), but free magnesium, as measured by magnetic resonance spectroscopy in the brain, is significantly less (.3–1 mM) (Vink et al. 1987, 1988).

There is a large family of G proteins, most of which are not well characterized. There are at least 20 different α subunits and four different β and δ subunits (Simon et al. 1991). Nonetheless, G proteins are generally classified as to whether they stimulate (G_s) or inhibit (G_i) adenylate cyclase, or whether they interact with phospholipase C (G_q or G_o).

Adenylate cyclase enzymes are equally as diverse. At least six types of the enzymes have been described, four of which are known to exist within the central nervous system (CNS) (W-J. Tang and Gilman 1991). Additionally, there are several forms of cyclic adenosine 3′, 5′ monophosphate (cAMP)-activated protein kinase (protein kinase A) (Walaas and Greengard 1991). Similarly, molecular cloning techniques have identified at least five distinct subtypes of phospholipase C (Bennett et al. 1988) and seven subtypes of its downstream protein kinase (protein kinase C) (see Figure 5–1) (Nishizuka 1988). This tremendous heterogeneity allows for a wide spectrum of cellular responses to a finite number of neurotransmitters.

ADENYLATE CYCLASE

Neurotransmitters can either activate adenylate cyclase (e.g., dopamine via D_1 [Kebabian and Calne 1979] or norepinephrine via β-adrenoceptors [Cassel and Selinger 1978; Schramm and Selinger 1984]) or inhibit adenylate cyclase (e.g., dopamine via D_2 [D. M. F. Cooper et al. 1986] or acetylcholine via M_2 [Akiyam et al. 1986; Olianas et al. 1983]) (Figure 5–1). Activation is mediated by the free α subunit of the G_s protein and results in the formation of cAMP from adenosine triphosphate (ATP) (Figure 5–1). cAMP binds to any of the two cAMP binding sites on each of the two regulatory (R) subunits of the inactive tetramer form of protein kinase A (Walaas and Greengard 1991). Binding of cAMP to these sites allows the two catalytic (C) subunits to dissociate from the R subunits and become active (Walaas and Greengard 1991). The active protein kinase A catalytic subunit can phosphorylate a wide variety of substrates, including voltage-sensitive calcium channels (Osterrieder et al. 1982), voltage-sensitive potassium channels (Castellucci et al. 1980; Osterrieder et al. 1982; Siegelbaum et al. 1982), voltage-sensitive sodium channels (Costa and Catterall 1984a; Costa et al. 1982), the inositol 1,4,5-triphosphate (IP_3) receptor (Supattapone et al. 1988), and various other proteins such as tyrosine hydroxylase, the nicotinic acetylcholine receptor, the β-adrenoceptor, and others (Nairn et al. 1985).

Inactivation of protein kinase A or reversal of its effects is mediated through at least four routes:

1. Hydrolysis of cAMP by a cyclic nucleotide phosphodiesterase will allow the R and C subunits to reassociate into the inactive tetramer form of the enzyme (Walaas and Greengard 1991).
2. Many tissues appear to possess a protein inhibitor that binds with and inactivates the C subunit (Ashby and Walsh 1972; Walsh et al. 1971). These proteins have primary structures that are quite similar to the phosphorylation sites of the actual physiological substrate phosphoproteins and are consequently called *pseudosubstrate prototypes*. Binding of the pseudosubstrate to the C subunit will inactivate the protein kinase; similarly, removal of the pseudosubstrate activates the kinase (Kemp and Pearson 1990; Kemp et al. 1975; Soderling 1990).

3. Phosphoprotein phosphates will dephosphorylate the proteins phosphorylated by the protein kinase and therefore work to return the system to its basal state (Walaas and Greengard 1991).
4. G_i may prevent the activation of the G_s protein. The mechanism by which G_i inhibits G_s is unknown. However, because G_i is present at greater concentrations than G_s (Neer et al. 1984), one model argues that $\beta\delta$ subunits released when G_i is activated bind to the α subunit of G_s, preventing it from stimulating adenylate cyclase (Baraban et al. 1989).

PHOSPHATIDYLINOSITOL SYSTEM

The PI second-messenger system is more complicated because one neurotransmitter or receptor agonist activates two second messengers (Figure 5–1). Activation of PI-linked G protein (G_o), in the presence of GTP and magnesium results in the activation of the membrane enzyme phospholipase C. Phospholipase C hydrolyzes both phosphatidylinositol 4 phosphate (PIP) and phosphatidylinositol 4,5-bisphosphate (PIP$_2$) to produce the second messengers diacylglycerol (DAG) and inositol 1,4,5-triphosphate (IP$_3$) (Figures 5–1 and 5–3) (Berridge 1984).

IP$_3$ stimulates the release of calcium from intracellular stores in the endoplasmic reticulum (Daniell and Harris 1989; Gandhi and Ross 1987; Joseph and Rice 1989; C. A. Ross et al. 1989; Stauderman et al. 1988) or specialized calcium-containing "calciosomes" (Volpe et al. 1988), resulting in a transient increase in intracellular free calcium. Sustained stimulation of the system that may occur under certain experimental conditions (e.g., using inositol 1,4,5-trisphosphorothioate [IP(s)$_3$], a nondegradable analogue of IP$_3$ [Taylor et al. 1989]) will deplete these intracellular calcium stores within 10–20 seconds and increase the influx of extracellular calcium (C. A. Hansen et al. 1990).

The IP$_3$ receptor is a glycoprotein composed of four subunits, with a molecular weight of approximately 300 kDa each (Fisher et al. 1991). Each unit has a single IP$_3$ binding site, and the binding of three or four IP$_3$ molecules will result in the opening of a central transmembrane calcium pore (Maeda et al. 1991; Meyer et al. 1988). In the CNS, IP$_3$ receptors are generally believed to be intracellular (Fisher et al. 1991), but there is evidence that in other tissues, such

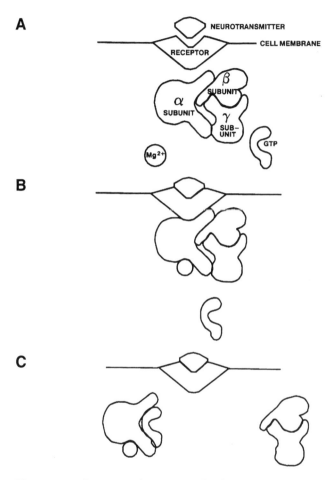

Figure 5–3.   Sequence of events involved in transduction of first-message signal to second messenger. *A:* At rest, the inactive G protein complex is composed of the three subunits α, β, γ. *B:* When the receptor is activated, and in the presence of magnesium and GTP, it interacts with the G protein complex to decrease affinity of the βγ units to the α subunit and to increase affinity of the α subunit to GTP. *C:* GTP binds to the α subunit, displacing the βγ subunits. The α subunit/GTP/magnesium complex is the activated form of the G protein and can activate such effectors as adenylate cyclase or phospholipase C. The α subunit self-inactivates by hydrolyzing GTP to GDP, thereby allowing the βγ subunits to reassociate to form the inactive αβγ complex.

as lymphocytes (A. A. Khan et al. 1992), the IP_3 receptors may be localized to the plasma membrane. The increase in free intracellular calcium may have direct effects (such as an increase in potassium conductance that results in a more negative resting potential and the after-hyperpolarization that follows action-potential bursts [McCarren et al. 1989; Pennefeather et al. 1985]) or indirect effects via calcium/calmodulin-dependent protein kinases (Walaas and Greengard 1991). Calcium/calmodulin kinase II has a wide range of substrate phosphoproteins, such as protein phosphatase 2BC (which dephosphorylates some of the proteins phosphorylated by the kinases), tyrosine hydroxylase, glycogen synthase, myelin basic protein, synapsin I, and others (Walaas and Greengard 1991). Although increases in intracellular free calcium are usually rapidly and efficiently terminated (Blaustein et al. 1980; Carafoli and Crompton 1978; Janis et al. 1987; Vincenzi and Larsen 1980), calcium/calmodulin kinase II possesses the ability to self-phosphorylate and liberate itself from dependence on either calcium or calmodulin (Fukunaga et al. 1989; Lai et al. 1986; Lou et al. 1986; Miller and Kennedy 1986; T. Saitoh and Schwartz 1985). This independence may allow calcium/calmodulin kinase II to remain active for a period of time beyond the normalization of intracellular calcium levels, but the enzyme is eventually inactivated by protein phosphatases (Y. Saitoh et al. 1987; Shields et al. 1985).

The original IP_3 signal is terminated quickly via hydrolysis by IP_3 phosphatase to inositol 1,4-biphosphate (IP_2) (Ragan 1990) or by phosphorylation to inositol 1,3,4,5-tetrakisphosphate (IP_4) (Figure 5–3). Specific, high-affinity receptors for IP_4 have recently been identified (Reiser et al. 1991), and this IP_3 metabolite may play a role in inducing calcium sequestration by the endoplasmic reticulum (T. D. Hill et al. 1988).

DAG is the other second messenger generated through the receptor-activated hydrolysis of PIP_2 by phospholipase C (Figure 5–1). However, although the only source of IP_3 is the hydrolysis of PIP_2, DAG may arise from the hydrolysis of PI, PIP, PIP_2 (Figure 5–3) (Berridge 1987; Downes 1982; Fisher and Agranoff 1987; Hill et al. 1988), phosphatidylcholine (Billah and Anthes 1990), and other inositol-containing glycolipids (Saltiel et al. 1986). Furthermore, because PIP concentration usually exceeds that of PIP_2 in the membrane, DAG production may be favored. This is seen in the cortex, striatum, and spinal cord, where the concentration of DAG-activated protein kinase C may greatly exceed the concentration of IP_3 (Baraban et al. 1989).

DAG is a neutral lipid and consequently remains within the membrane (Bruzzone 1990). Protein kinase C is a cytoplasmic enzyme that is believed to migrate toward the membrane when intracellular calcium is increased (Baraban et al. 1989). Nonetheless, DAG activates protein kinase C by increasing its sensitivity to calcium and can thus activate the enzyme in the absence of changes in intracellular calcium concentrations (Bruzzone 1990). The activated protein kinase C, in turn, phosphorylates a wide range of phosphoprotein substrates, including the sodium channel (Costa and Catterall 1984b), calcium channel (Albert et al. 1984), IP_3 phosphatase (Baraban et al. 1989), tyrosine hydroxylase (Albert et al. 1984), myelin basic protein, and others (Walaas and Greengard 1991).

Phosphorylation of IP_3 phosphatase by protein kinase C activates it and accelerates the rate of IP_3 breakdown, thereby decreasing the magnitude of calcium released from intracellular stores (Baraban et al. 1989). This action counters the tendency toward hyperpolarization caused by the calcium-activated potassium current (McCarren et al. 1989; Pennefeather et al. 1985; Sawada et al. 1989) and increases both neuronal excitability (Baraban et al. 1985) and neurotransmitter release (Nichols et al. 1987; Shapira et al. 1987; Zurgil et al. 1986).

DAG is inactivated by phosphorylation by DAG kinase into phosphatidic acid (Figure 5–3) (Berridge 1984). Actions of protein kinase C are terminated by phosphoprotein phosphatases (Walaas and Greengard 1991) or inactivation by pseudosubstrate prototypes (House and Kemp 1987; Kemp et al. 1989).

Once formed, the second messengers IP_3 and DAG are recycled to form more membrane phosphatidylinositol (Figure 5–3). IP_3 is eventually metabolized to inositol monophosphate (IP_1) (any one of at least three isomers with phosphate group at the 1, 3, or 4 position). IP_1 is hydrolyzed by IP_1 phosphatase to produce free inositol (Figure 5–3). Inositol and the DAG metabolite cytidine diphosphate-diacylglycerol (CDP-DAG) form PI, which gives rise to PIP and PIP_2 via PI kinase and PIP kinase, respectively (Figure 5–3) (Berridge 1984).

G PROTEIN FUNCTION IN BIPOLAR ILLNESS

Avissar and Schreiber (1989) propounded that the acetylcholine-linked G protein system is hyperfunctional in both ill phases of bipolar illness. This hypothesis is supported by a study conducted by Schreiber et al. (1991), who looked at the increase in Gpp(NH)p (a nonhydrolyzable analogue of GTP with a higher affinity to G protein) resulting from isoproterenol and carbamylcholine treatment of mononuclear cells obtained from patients and control subjects. They studied 10 acutely manic patients who had been unmedicated for at least 1 month; 10 euthymic, lithium-treated patients; and 10 matched mental health staff as control subjects. Maximal binding of GTP or Gpp(NH)p to G protein in response to both isoproterenol and carbamylcholine was increased in the acutely manic individuals ($P < .001$ for both) but normal in lithium-treated euthymic patients.

SITE OF LITHIUM ACTION: G PROTEINS

Early investigators noted increased urinary excretion of cAMP in manic patients (Abdulla and Hamadah 1970; Paul et al. 1970a, 1970b). Subsequent observations that β adrenoceptor agonists elevate plasma cAMP (Ball et al. 1972) and that lithium prevents agonist-induced adenylate cyclase activity in animals (Ebstein et al. 1980; Forn and Valdecasas 1971; Newman et al. 1985; Walker 1974) and in bipolar patients (Ebstein et al. 1976) supported the belief that lithium antagonizes a noradrenergic hyperactivity in mania. More recent reports, particularly by Belmaker, Schreiber, Avissar, and their colleagues, have suggested that lithium exerts these actions by antagonizing agonist-stimulated GTP binding to the α subunit of G proteins (Avissar and Schreiber 1989; Avissar et al. 1988).

This model proposes that lithium competes with magnesium at the low-affinity magnesium binding site needed for $\beta\delta$ subunit complex-GTP exchange (Figure 5–2) (Avissar et al. 1991). By doing so, lithium decreases the ability of all neurotransmitters using G proteins to produce a second messenger. By reducing the transducing ability of G proteins, lithium can attenuate a wide variety of hyperactive neurotransmitter and neuromodulator signals that may be present in mania.

Experimental Evidence

Early in vitro studies examining the effect of lithium on cAMP accumulation usually were conducted using toxic levels of lithium (≥ 2 mM) (Forn and Valdecasas 1971; Walker 1974), leading some authors to argue that these outcomes bore no relationship to the therapeutic actions of lithium. However, more careful studies by Belmaker and his associates clearly showed that lithium has these effects at therapeutic ranges both in vitro (Ebstein et al. 1980; Newman et al. 1985) and in vivo in humans (Ebstein et al. 1976). Furthermore, there is evidence that lithium antagonizes many, if not all, neurotransmitters linked with adenylate cyclase via G proteins, including norepinephrine, acetylcholine (Avissar and Schreiber 1989; Avissar et al. 1991), serotonin (Mork and Geisler 1989), thyrotropin-stimulating hormone (Wolff et al. 1970), prostaglandins (Wang et al. 1974), and forskolin, which is a plant alkaloid that is a potent activator of adenylate cyclase (Andersen and Geisler 1984; Andersen et al. 1984; Newman and Belmaker 1987).

That lithium toxicity may result secondarily to extensive inhibition of adenylate cyclase was tested by the acute administration of high doses of lithium and the adenylate cyclase stimulator forskolin (Belmaker et al. 1981). Forskolin did not prevent or delay lithium-induced death, suggesting that this may not be the mechanism of lithium toxicity (Belmaker et al. 1981).

Lithium's interaction with magnesium at the low-affinity magnesium binding site of the G protein appears to be somewhat specific. Lithium does not interfere with the high-affinity magnesium binding site required for GTPase activity (Fleming and Watanabe 1988; G. Hill and Jacobs 1989). Furthermore, although lithium inhibition of GTP binding is evident at physiological magnesium concentrations, it can be overridden by supraphysiological magnesium concentrations (5 mM) (Avissar et al. 1991). This suggests that a possible role for magnesium is ameliorating lithium toxicity; however, although there is one such case report (Worthley 1974), more extensive evidence is lacking. Additionally, the ability of lithium to uncouple G protein transduction has not been replicated (Ellis and Lenox 1991).

Variations in the structure and distribution of G protein subunits may help explain some of the CNS selectivity of lithium. For example, lithium inhibition of isoproterenol-induced GTP binding in the brain, but not in the heart (Schreiber et al. 1990), may be partially caused by the observation that the predominant form of the α subunit of G protein in the brain is a 50-kDa protein, whereas the heart mainly contains a 45-kDa form (Mumby et al. 1986).

PHOSPHATIDYLINOSITOL IN BIPOLAR ILLNESS

Despite the flurry of basic investigation, clinical work in this area is relatively scarce. Sengupta et al. (1981) measured platelet and erythrocyte membrane phospholipids in 22 medicated and 21 medication-free bipolar patients. They found significant reductions in membrane phosphatidylcholine, phosphatidylserine, and phosphatidylethanolamine but no differences in PI (Sengupta et al. 1981).

Conversely, Kato et al. (1991), using ^{31}P magnetic resonance spectroscopy to measure phosphorus metabolism in vivo, found that the phosphomonoester peak (which is reflective of many kinds of sugar phosphates, phosphoethanolamine, and phosphocholine [Gyulai et al. 1984; Hope et al. 1984]) was elevated during acute mania compared with euthymia in lithium-treated patients (Kato et al. 1991). In one patient studied before initiating lithium therapy, the initiation of lithium was associated with an increase in the phosphomonoester peak, which subsequently decreased with recovery of mood despite the continuation of lithium therapy (Kato et al. 1991). Because the phosphomonoester peak measured a variety of phoso-compounds, it is very difficult to interpret this data.

Belmaker et al. (1990a) measured inositol monophosphatase activity in red blood cells obtained from medication-free manic patients, lithium-treated manic patients, and normal drug-free control subjects. At a mean lithium level of 0.52 mM, there was a 78% decrease in enzyme activity. Unmedicated manic patients did not differ from control subjects.

Banks et al. (1990), measured [³H]-inositol incorporation into lymphoblastoid cells established from bipolar patients and control subjects. Although inositol uptake and intracellular levels were similar, cells derived from bipolar patients incorporated 50%–60% less [³H]-inositol into phospholipids after 6 hours.

SITE OF LITHIUM ACTION: INOSITOL MONOPHOSPHATASE

Although lithium was first demonstrated to influence inositol metabolism as early as 1971 (Allison and Stewart), it was not until 1982, following reports of specific lithium inhibition of inositol monophosphatase (Hallcher and Sherman 1980), that Berridge et al. (1982) proposed that this may be the site of clinical action of lithium. According to this model, lithium's ability to inhibit inositol monophosphatase causes a relative depletion of free inositol and a consequent depletion of PIP_2 formation (See Figure 5–3). Furthermore, because lithium's action is uncompetitive, the magnitude of lithium's effect would be expected to be proportional to the level of PIP_2 hydrolysis (Nahorski et al. 1991; Ragan 1990). That is, at low levels of neurotransmitter-induced PIP_2 hydrolysis, the effect of lithium on the system would be minimal and easily overcome. However, as neurotransmitter-induced second-messenger generation is increased, lithium would significantly interfere with the system. Consequently, the model suggests that under normal physiological conditions, the effect of lithium would be minimal, but as neurotransmitter turnover increases, as would be expected in mania and perhaps depression, lithium interferes with the second-messenger response.

The model also explains why the effects of lithium, particularly at toxic levels (El-Mallakh 1986a), are primarily central. Inositol is plentiful in the diet and all body tissues. Its intracellular concentration may be 100 times greater than the plasma concentration of .1 mM (Hauser 1969; Spector 1976; Spector and Lorenzo 1975). Although peripheral tissues can readily access plasma inositol, transport into the CNS occurs via a saturable mechanism (Spector and

Lorenzo 1975). This normally limits the fraction of cerebrospinal fluid inositol derived from plasma to 2% (Barkai 1981; Margolis et al. 1971). Brain inositol probably originates from de novo synthesis from glucose-6-phosphate to form inositol (3) monophosphate. However, inositol (3) monophosphate must be hydrolyzed by the lithium-sensitive inositol monophosphatase to produce free inositol (Figure 5–3) (Nahorski et al. 1991). Consequently, lithium both blocks the recycling of inositol and prevents its de novo synthesis. Thus, the brain's unique dependence on local de novo inositol synthesis makes it more susceptible to lithium's effect.

Experimental Evidence

Although initial data strongly supported the inositol monophosphatase model of lithium action, a subsequent lack of reproducibility and an incomplete understanding of IP metabolism have tempered enthusiasm. Allison and Stewart (1971) were the first to report that acute intraperitoneal injections of lithium chloride (10 mEq/kg body weight) caused a significant (> 30%) decrease of basal rat brain myoinositol levels (Allison and Blisner 1976; Allison and Stewart 1971; Hirvonen 1991; Ragan et al. 1988). Subsequently, some researchers showed that this decrease is associated with a large increase in inositol (1) monophosphate (IP_1) (Allison et al. 1976; Honchar et al. 1983; Sherman et al. 1981; Whitworth et al. 1990), whereas others found no changes in basal IP_1 levels (Godfrey et al. 1989; Kendall and Nahorski 1987; Li et al. 1993). As suggested by Li et al. (1993), these differences may be related to different levels of lithium achieved by the different investigators.

Chronic lithium administration, which produces more comparable serum lithium levels, results in a reproducible increase in basal IP_1 accumulation (Honchar et al. 1990; Kendall and Nahorski 1987; Li et al. 1993; Sherman et al. 1985, 1986). Interestingly, despite reports to the contrary (Renshaw et al. 1986), there do not appear to be compensatory changes in inositol monophosphatase activity (Honchar et al. 1989, 1990; Nahorski et al. 1991; Sherman et al. 1985, 1986).

Because lithium appears to inhibit inositol monophosphatase activity via an uncompetitive mechanism, the potency of which is related to the activity of the system (Nahorski et al. 1991; Ragan 1990), its effect would be expected to be magnified when the system is activated. This is clearly seen in acute studies where coadministration of lithium and muscarinic agonists (e.g., pilocarpine) can cause a tenfold increase in IP_1 and can produce seizures and brain damage (Honchar et al. 1983; Whitworth et al. 1990). This effect can be blocked by anticholinergics such as atropine (Honchar et al. 1983; Whitworth et al. 1990).

On the other hand, chronic lithium treatment (2 weeks) appears to decrease agonist-stimulated (carbachol or norepinephrine) PIP_2 hydrolysis as measured by IP_1 accumulation (Casebolt and Jope 1987; Kendall and Nahorski 1987; Li et al. 1993; Whitworth and Kendall 1989). This would be expected if chronic lithium treatment prevented PIP_2 repletion by depleting inositol (Figure 5–3). Although chronic lithium treatment does not reduce total levels of PI, PIP, or PIP_2 (Honchar et al. 1989; Sherman et al. 1985), the existence of receptor-specific pools that may be susceptible to depletion has been proposed by various researchers (Cubitt et al. 1990; Whitworth and Kendall 1989; Yorek et al. 1991a).

Additional evidence that lithium may act via the inhibition of inositol formation comes from studies documenting a reversal of lithium-induced neurotoxicity with myoinositol. Although orally administered, myoinositol is ineffectual in preventing lithium-toxicity-induced death (Belmaker et al. 1990a) or behavioral changes (Belmaker et al. 1990b). Intracranially administered myoinositol reversed the lithium-induced inhibition of rearing (Kofman and Belmaker 1990) and antagonized the epileptogenic combination of lithium and pilocarpine in rats (Tricklebank et al. 1991). These observations also provide support for the relative inaccessibility to the brain of systemically available inositol.

Although not well investigated, lithium does affect the DAG arm of the phospholipase C second-messenger system. DAG and its metabolites CMP-PA and CDP-DAG (see Figure 5–3) are elevated by lithium in cortical slices in vitro (Drummond and Raeburn 1984; Godfrey 1989; Kennedy et al. 1990). This elevation is presumed to occur because of the reduced incorporation of CDP-DAG into PI resulting from free-inositol deficiency. This supposition is supported by observations that inositol can reverse lithium's effect on DAG in vitro (Watson et al. 1990) and in embryogenesis ex vivo (Busa and Gimlich 1989). In rats, chronic lithium treatment does not appear to alter either the distribution or the activity of the DAG-dependent protein kinase C (Casebolt and Jope 1991) but does alter protein kinase C–mediated phosphorylation (Casebolt and Jope 1991), reduces its major substrate (the "MARCKS" protein for myristoylated alanine-rich C kinase substrate [Lenox and Watson 1994; Manji et al. 1995]), and affects several other phosphoproteins (Casebolt and Jope 1991; Klein et al. 1987; Vatal and Aiyar 1984). Understanding the potential effects of lithium in terms of protein phosphorylation is currently not possible for several reasons: the function of many of these phosphoproteins is still unknown; some phosphoproteins may be susceptible to phosphorylation by different protein kinases (Walaas and Greengard 1991); and lithium can, either directly or indirectly, alter the activity of at least three different protein kinases.

SUMMARY

Lithium has significant effects on message-transducing G proteins and the phosphatidylinositol second-messenger system. The latter is linked to a wide array of neuropeptides and neurotransmitters, including norepinephrine via α_1 receptors, acetylcholine via the muscarinic type of receptors, serotonin via 5-HT$_{1c}$ and 5-HT$_2$, histamine via H$_1$, and glutamate via the quisqualate type of receptors (Nahorski 1988). These effects occur at therapeutic lithium levels and are always in the direction of decreasing signal intensity. Thus, lithium appears to interfere with the activity of a range of neurotransmitters that may have excitatory or inhibitory action. This range of action suggests that the effects of lithium, and probably the pathophysiological abnormality of bipolar illness itself, may be more universal in nature than was previously thought; that is, they are probably not limited to a unique neurotransmitter system.

Chapter 6

Ionic Mechanisms
of Lithium Action

In classic pharmacology, one often attempts to identify ligand or receptor binding sites as an initial step in unraveling mechanisms of action. For lithium, an ion in aqueous solutions, the major receptor site is ion pumps and channels. Consequently, regardless of what lithium may do to first or second messengers, an investigation into how it may interact with ion channels is essential in understanding its mechanisms of action. What makes this line of investigation essential is the fact that mood-disordered states themselves are characterized by changes in fluid and ion balance.

ION CONTROL AND NEURONAL ACTIVITY

A high degree of ion regulation is essential for proper neuronal activity. At the heart of these processes is the sodium- and potassium-activated adenosine triphosphatase (Na,K-ATPase) pump. This membrane pump uses energy in the form of adenosine triphosphate (ATP) to pump out three sodium ions in exchange for two potassium ions (Eisner and Lederer 1980; Lederer and Nelson 1984; Rakowski et al. 1989; Sen and Post 1964). By creating an electrochemical gradient of sodium and potassium ions, the pump generates a potential difference across the membrane. The relative impermeability of the membrane to sodium creates a membrane capacitance that is used to generate the current of the action potential.

The Na,K-ATPase enzyme is composed of two protein subunits (Figure 6–1). A large catalytic subunit (α) possesses all the functions and properties ascribed to Na,K-ATPase (i.e., ion, ouabain, and ATP binding sites) (Horisberger et al. 1991). A smaller glyco-

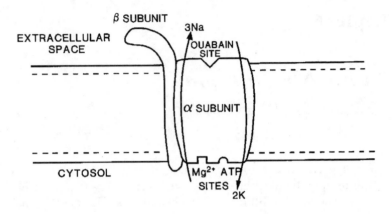

Figure 6–1. Schematic representation of the structure of the Na,K-ATPase showing the α and β subunits and the active pump and ligand sites. *Source.* Reprinted from El-Mallakh and Li 1993. Used with permission.

protein, the β subunit, is required for functionally active Na,K-ATPase (Noguchi et al. 1987; Takeda et al. 1988) and may play an essential role in anchoring newly synthesized α subunits (Hiatt et al. 1984). There are at least three loci for the α subunit (α_1, α_2, α_3) (Berrebi-Bertrand et al. 1990; Urayama et al. 1989) and probably three for the β subunit as well (β_1, β_2, β_3) (Horisberger et al. 1991). Alpha subunits are highly conserved through evolution ($\geq 90\%$ nucleotide identity from drosophila fruit flies to humans), whereas the β subunit is less conserved across taxonomic classes (60% identity) (Horisberger et al. 1991). The three α isoforms probably arose from one ancestral form and share 80%–86% of the base sequences. The predominant form in the kidney and in early brain development is α_1. It is distinguished from α_2 and α_3 by having a lower affinity for ouabain, and α_2 is the most sensitive to inhibition by ouabain (IC_{50} 23 nM, 460 nM, and 320,000 nM ouabain for α_2, α_3, and α_1, respectively) (Berrebi-Bertrand et al. 1990).

In rat brains, α_2 and α_3 begin to replace α_1 during the last week of gestation and increase rapidly thereafter (Atterwill and Collins 1987; Schmitt and McDonough 1986; Specht 1984). The increase in α_2 and α_3 is accompanied by large ionic shifts (Valcana and Timiras

1969; Vernadakis and Woodbury 1962) and the appearance of electroencephalographic activity (Abdel-Latif et al. 1967). Results from mRNA Northern Blot analysis of tissue culture cells suggest that α_2 is predominant in glia and α_3, in neurons (Corthesy-Theulaz et al. 1990); α_3 may be most prominent in axons, but cell bodies contain both α_2 and α_3 (Sweadner 1991). Interestingly, although high ouabain affinity Na,K-ATPase is responsible for 80% of total ATP cleaving activity in synaptosomes, it accounts for only 27% of total sodium movement across the resting membrane. This differential indicates that resting neuronal membranes use only 1.4% of possible high ouabain affinity Na,K-ATPase (Brodsky and Guidotti 1990). Nonetheless, this characteristic results in extraordinary gradients of < 20 mM intracellular sodium ions versus > 130 mM extracellular sodium ions and > 140 mM intracellular potassium ions versus < 10 mM potassium ions in the extracellular fluid (Civan and Shporer 1989). Because of the large concentration of impermeable intracellular anions, the result is a neuronal resting potential close to the potassium potential of –75 mV.

An excitatory neurotransmitter interacting with the dendritic membrane will increase sodium influx and produce an excitatory postsynaptic potential (usually around 120–240 µV) (Figure 6–2). The sum of several such potentials (approximately 700 µV) will produce an action potential at the axonal hillock that will self-propagate to the presynaptic terminal (Figure 6–2) (Hodgkin 1964; Kuffler and Nicholl 1979).

At the presynaptic terminal, sodium influx results in a short-lived increase of free ionic calcium from 10^{-7} M to the physiologically active range between 10^{-7}M and 10^{-6}M (Figure 6–2) (Janis et al. 1987). This so-called *calcium transient* brings about neurotransmitter release (Katz and Miledi 1967b; Miledi 1973; Zucker and Lando 1986). Neuronal presynaptic terminals are unique among excitable tissues in that they rely on extracellular calcium—not intracellular stores—to produce the calcium transient (Baker 1972; Blaustein 1974; Katz and Miledi 1967a, 1967b, 1967c). Extracellular calcium may enter via sodium-calcium counterexchange (three intracellular sodium ions exchanged for one extracellular calcium ion [Baker et al. 1969; Blaustein 1974; Blaustein and Wiesmann 1970; Blaustein et al. 1974; Carafoli and Longoni 1987; Racker 1980]) or

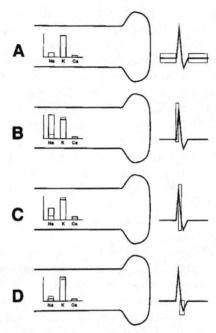

Figure 6–2.   Schematic representation of changes in intracellular sodium, potassium, and calcium concentrations during an action potential. **A**: At rest, intraneuronal potassium concentration is quite high ($\sim$10^{-4} mM). **B**: Depolarization of the membrane during an action potential is caused by rapid sodium influx. **C**: Several mechanisms attempt to compensate for the sudden elevation of intracellular sodium content; these include the Na,K-ATPase, potassium efflux, and sodium-calcium counterexchange. At the presynaptic nerve terminal, the small, transient increase in free calcium ion concentration may bring about neurotransmitter release. **D**: Recovery from the action potential is usually accompanied by excessive sodium efflux and a brief transient membrane hyperpolarization. The free ionic calcium transient is eliminated by a variety of mechanisms, and neurotransmitter release is terminated.
Source.   Reprinted from El-Mallakh and Li 1993. Used with permission.

through voltage-dependent calcium channels (Smith and Augustine 1988). Thus, it is not surprising that the number of quanta of neurotransmitters released per impulse is directly proportional to the amplitude of the action potential (Martin 1966).

Because of the extraordinary biological activity of free ionic calcium, calcium buffering in neurons must be efficient. Calcium binds to cytoplasmic proteins and is taken up by endoplasmic reticula or mitochondria or is extruded from the cell (Figure 6–2) (Blaustein 1988; Blaustein et al. 1980; Carafoli and Crompton 1978; Vincenzi and Larsen 1980). Bulk calcium extrusion is accomplished by high-capacity, low-affinity sodium-calcium counterexchange (Baker et al. 1969; Blaustein 1974, 1988; Blaustein and Wiesmann 1970; Blaustein et al. 1974, 1980; Carafoli and Longoni 1987; Racker 1980), whereas fine-tuning of the intracellular calcium concentration requires the low-capacity, high-affinity calcium-activated, magnesium-dependent ATPase (Carafoli and Longoni 1987; Robinson 1981).

ION BALANCE AND BIPOLAR ILLNESS

Beginning in the 1940s and continuing into the 1950s, investigators noted mood-state–related alterations in fluid and electrolyte balance (Klein et al. 1945; Schottstaedt et al. 1956a, 1956b, 1956c). Subsequently, Coppen and Shaw studied the fluid compartment distribution of ^{24}sodium and ^{82}bromine in both of the ill phases of bipolar disorder (Coppen et al. 1966; Shaw 1966) and in unipolar depression (Coppen and Shaw 1963). They found that residual sodium (defined as the intracellular sodium plus a small amount of readily exchangeable bone sodium) is increased in both mania and depression and that it returns to normal upon recovery. Naylor et al. (1970) also found a statistically significant increase in intraerythrocyte sodium in two studies composed of 44 severely depressed women (both unipolar and bipolar) compared before and after recovery. A group of 29 "neurotically" depressed women did not exhibit any sodium changes. All of these women were studied on a "metabolic unit" under conditions of strict control of caloric and salt intake, and all were unmedicated at least 4 days before samples were obtained (Naylor et al. 1970). Baer et al. (1970a) reported a similar trend in four bipolar patients, but Mendels et al. (1972a) found intraerythrocyte sodium to be lower in 10 ill bipolar patients and that it did not vary with recovery.

Because relative sodium concentrations across cellular membranes are determined chiefly by Na,K-ATPase activity, this early work led to a series of investigations, spanning some 20 years, of

Na,K-ATPase activity in mood disorders (Akagawa et al. 1980; D. R. Alexander et al. 1986; Choi et al. 1977; Hesketh 1976; Hesketh et al. 1977, 1978; Hokin-Neaverson and Jefferson 1989a, 1989b; Hokin-Neaverson et al. 1974, 1976; Johnston et al. 1980; Linnoila et al. 1983; Naylor and Smith 1981; Naylor et al. 1973, 1976a, 1976b, 1980; Nurnberger et al. 1982; Reddy et al. 1989, 1992; Rybakowski et al. 1981; Scott and Reading 1978; Sengupta et al. 1980; Thakar et al. 1985; Whalley et al. 1980; Wood et al. 1989). Recently, this extensive literature was critically reviewed by S. W. Looney and El-Mallakh (unpublished data, March 1995); we also conducted a meta-analysis to determine the nature of Na,K-ATPase changes in bipolar illness. Bipolar depressed individuals (Figure 6–3, A) and manic individuals (Figure 6–3, B) were found to have significantly lower Na,K-ATPase activity when compared with recovered individuals but not when compared with normal control subjects (Figure 6–3, C). The effect size was nonsignificantly greater in depression (0.62) than in mania (0.42) and was moderate for both states. These findings are quite compatible with the previously presented Na,K-ATPase hypothesis for bipolar illness (El-Mallakh 1983a; El-Mallakh et al. 1993). Within the framework of this hypothesis, a modest decrease in pump activity produces mania, whereas a more significant decrease brings about depression.

Calcium regulation is also altered as a function of mood in bipolar illness. Dubovsky et al. (1989, 1991, 1992) have consistently found mood-state–related increases in intracellular calcium in bipolar patients. This increase is an expected consequence of decreased sodium pump activity and increased intracellular sodium (El-Mallakh and Jaziri 1990). Specifically, an increase in intracellular sodium slows intracellular calcium clearance by the sodium-calcium counterexchange system (see above). Although the unavailability of a specific sodium-calcium counterexchange inhibitor prevents direct study of this pump, investigators have reported abnormalities of the magnesium-sensitive Ca-ATPase pump (Meltzer and Kassir 1983). Interestingly, the activity of this system tends to be nonsignificantly lower in bipolar manic patients (Scott and Reading 1978) and bipolar depressed patients (Choi et al. 1977; Rybakowski et al. 1981) than in either healthy control subjects or recovered bipolar patients. In addition, a small number of studies

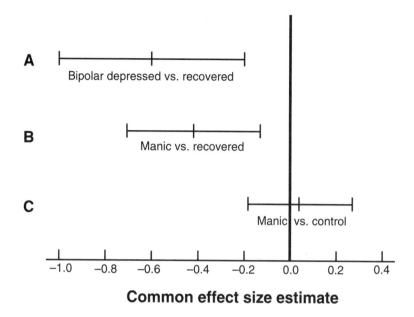

Common effect size estimate

Figure 6–3. Results of meta-analysis of studies of erythrocyte Na,K-ATPase activity as a function of the various moods of bipolar illness. The bars give the mean effect size and 95% confidence limits for the noted comparisons. (If the effect size bar spans 0, it is not significant.)

examining a small number of patients also failed to find a difference (Linnoila et al. 1983; Whalley et al. 1980). Unfortunately, the size of the literature is inadequate to allow us to perform a meta-analysis (discussed earlier regarding the sodium pump). Nonetheless, some investigators believe that this abnormality may play a direct role in the pathogenesis of bipolar illness (Dubovsky and Franks 1983).

THE NA,K-ATPASE HYPOTHESIS FOR BIPOLAR ILLNESS

The findings of mood-state–related alterations in ionic control have led to several ionic models of the illness (El-Mallakh 1983a; El-Mallakh et al. 1993; Meltzer 1993; Naylor et al. 1987; Singh 1970).

One of the better developed models is the Na,K-ATPase hypothesis for bipolar illness (Figure 6–4) (El-Mallakh 1983a; El-Mallakh and Wyatt 1995; El-Mallakh et al. 1993; Singh 1970). This hypothesis states that both mania and bipolar depression result from a unidirectional decrease in Na,K-ATPase activity. This decrease is believed to be universal (i.e., equally affecting all cells of the body) but relatively small. However, neurons, because of their extreme dependence on proper sodium pump activity, may exhibit the greatest functional effects.

Specifically, as Na,K-ATPase activity begins to fall, neuronal transmembrane resting potential begins to approach threshold potential (Figure 6–4), which may make the neuron more irritable. Additionally, the resulting increase in intracellular cationic sodium accumulation will decrease the efficacy of hyperpolarizing inhibitory neurotransmitters. Finally, the increase in intracellular calcium that would result from sodium-calcium counterexchange may increase the quanta of neurotransmitters released with each action potential. That is, all the forces would act to increase neurotransmitter release and neuronal firing and to decrease inhibitory control, which is believed to result in mania (Figure 6–4).

As sodium pump activity continues to drop, however, some of the effects begin to change. Transmembrane resting potential continues to approach threshold, thereby further increasing neuronal irritability (Figure 6–4). However, the associated decrease in action potential amplitude (Hodgkin 1964) would result in a decrease of the number of quanta released per impulse (Martin 1966). If resting potential were equal to threshold potential, the neuron would become totally refractory (Figure 6–4). The greater intracellular positive change would be a greater hindrance to the action of inhibitory hyperpolarizing neurotransmitters, thereby greatly disrupting inhibitory neural control. Finally, the additional increase in intracellular calcium may result in a continuous subthreshold release of neurotransmitters and perhaps neurotransmitter depletion. These changes would result in mixed states and bipolar depression (Figure 6–4).

If the process continued such that the majority of neurons were at or above threshold, most brain activity could not be initiated or processed. This would result in catatonia. Thus, within the frame-

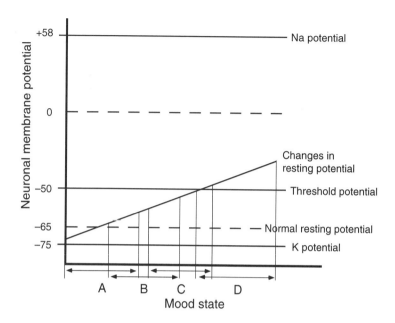

Figure 6–4. A schematic representation of the Na,K-ATPase hypothesis for bipolar illness. **A**: Represents the range of neuronal resting potentials of an ideal normal neuron. **B**: The range of resting potentials that may produce mania. **C**: The range of resting potentials that may produce bipolar depression. **D**: When the potential reaches or surpasses threshold, neurons become unresponsive. This may manifest as catatonia.
Source. El-Mallakh and Wyatt 1995. Used with permission.

work of the Na,K-ATPase hypothesis, mania is the milder form, depression the more severe form, and catatonia the severest form of the illness. The Na,K-ATPase hypothesis is a useful tool for understanding both bipolar illness and the various proposed modes of action of lithium (see Epilogue).

SITE OF LITHIUM ACTION: IONIC DISPLACEMENT

Lithium may traverse cellular membranes by any of four independent mechanisms: the sodium pump (sodium, potassium adenosine triphosphatase) (Figure 6–1), the sodium leak or spike channel, the sodium-lithium counterexchange system, and a lithium-bicarbonate anion exchange system (Ehrlich and Diamond 1979; Pandey et al. 1979). Under normal physiological conditions and at clinically relevant lithium concentrations, the sodium channel and sodium-lithium counterexchange systems are the most important (Ehrlich and Diamond 1979; El-Mallakh 1990a; Pandey et al. 1979).

The major route of lithium entry is the sodium channel. This is especially true for excitable tissues in which the opening of the sodium channel produces the action potential (El-Mallakh 1990a). The major route of lithium efflux is via the sodium-lithium counterexchange system. Whereas sodium-lithium counterexchange is potentially bidirectional, the direction of lithium movement is dependent on the sodium gradient across the membrane (Frazer et al. 1977; Lieberman et al. 1978; Swann et al. 1990). Specifically, lithium can be transported against its own concentration gradient toward the higher sodium concentration. In excitable tissues, the rate of lithium influx generally exceeds efflux. This manifests, in part, as a greater than twofold accumulation of lithium in the brains of lithium-treated animals (Heurteaux et al. 1986; Schmalzing 1986).

Intracellular lithium accumulation in human patients can be approximated by measuring the erythrocyte lithium ratio (expressed as the intraerythrocyte lithium concentration/plasma lithium concentration) (also see Chapter 1). The lithium ratio is determined by the balance of lithium influx via the sodium channel and lithium efflux via sodium-lithium counterexchange. In the erythrocyte, which maintains a membrane potential of approximately $-10V$ and is not excitable (Lassen 1972), the lithium ratio is determined primarily by the activity of sodium-lithium counterexchange (Ostrow et al. 1978). The activity of sodium-lithium counterexchange appears to be largely under genetic control (Dorus et al. 1983; Hasstedt et al. 1988), but despite reports to the contrary (Ostrow et al. 1978), it does not appear to be impaired in most bipolar patients (Dagher et al. 1984; Water et al. 1983). Nonetheless, most bipolar patients appear to have an elevated lithium ratio.

Lithium Ratio in Bipolar Individuals

Lithium-treated patients, regardless of diagnosis, will show an increase in their lithium ratio (Amsterdam et al. 1988; Ehrlich et al. 1979, 1981; Meltzer et al. 1977; Rybakowski et al. 1978a). This is believed to be a result of lithium-induced changes in sodium-lithium counterexchange and is detectable within 1–5 days of lithium treatment (Ehrlich et al. 1979, 1981). Interestingly, neuroleptic agents have similar effects (Albrect and Müller-Oerlinghausen 1976; Pandey et al. 1979). However, bipolar patients appear to have a higher lithium ratio, above and beyond this lithium effect. In four studies of 281 bipolar patients compared with 146 nonbipolar psychiatric patients and 56 healthy control subjects receiving lithium, the ratio was always significantly higher in bipolar patients than in the other comparison groups (Knorring et al. 1976; Ramsey et al. 1979a, 1979b; Rybakowski et al. 1978b; Szentistvány et al. 1980). Negative studies are few and usually have had small samples (Dagher et al. 1984; Ryan et al. 1989).

The increased lithium ratio observed in bipolar patients probably relates to alterations in sodium metabolism that are specific to bipolar illness (Coppen et al. 1966; Naylor et al. 1973; Shaw 1966). Bipolar illness is characterized by decreased Na,K-ATPase activity in both phases of the illness (see above and Figure 6–3), which probably underlies the observed retention of whole body and intracellular sodium by bipolar patients (see above) (Coppen et al. 1966; Naylor et al. 1973; D. M. Shaw 1966). Because the distribution of lithium is dependent on the relative sodium gradients (Frazer et al. 1977; Lieberman et al. 1978; Swann et al. 1990), it is not unexpected that acutely ill bipolar individuals retain more of the administered lithium than healthy control subjects (Almy and Taylor 1973), patients with personality disorders (Epstein et al. 1965), or euthymic bipolar patients (Greenspan et al. 1968a). Furthermore, the retained lithium is distributed in the extravascular (probably intracellular) compartments (Greenspan et al. 1968b) and would show up as a higher lithium ratio.

Lithium Ratio and Lithium Response

However, not all bipolar patients have a high lithium ratio. Some investigators have argued that the finding of an elevated lithium ratio is not random and holds implications regarding the treatment of bipolar illness. Specifically, many researchers have reported that the lithium ratio appears to be a predictor of therapeutic and prophylactic response to lithium treatment (see Chapter 1).

If the site of action of lithium is indeed intracellular, as is likely to be the case (see Epilogue), then one may argue that lithium response is related to the accumulation of "therapeutic intracellular levels of lithium," independent of serum lithium levels. Intuitively, such a conceptualization makes sense; intraerythrocyte lithium concentrations correlate much more closely with brain lithium levels than with plasma lithium levels in animals that were administered lithium acutely ($r = .95$ versus .46) and chronically ($r = .94$ versus .79) (Frazer et al. 1973). A similar pattern appears to exist in humans, with muscle lithium accumulation paralleling red blood cell levels more closely than plasma levels (Swann et al. 1990).

Intracellular Lithium Levels and Lithium Toxicity

The predictive power of intraerythrocyte lithium levels is perhaps best seen in studies of side effects or toxicity. In a study of 34 outpatients, the occurrence of side effects such as tremor and thirst was more strongly correlated with intraerythrocyte lithium levels ($r = .649$) than with either plasma levels ($r = .589$) or the lithium ratio ($r = .304$) (Albrect and Müller-Oerlinghausen 1976).

Similarly, of 77 patients on lithium, nine who experienced persistent side effects such as tremor, polyuria, and polydipsia had significantly higher intraerythrocyte lithium levels (mean = .33 mEq/L red blood cells) than the remaining individuals (mean = .24 mEq/L red blood cells, $P < .05$). Serum lithium levels were not significantly different (Hewick and Murray 1976).

Of 21 patients with normal prelithium electroencephalograms (EEGs), the 10 patients who developed abnormal EEG patterns had a significantly higher intraerythrocyte lithium concentration than the 11 patients with persistently normal EEGs (mean ± SD: .78 ± .20 versus .34 ± −.13 mEq/L red blood cells, $P < .01$). Serum lithium levels were higher in the abnormal EEG group, but the difference was not significant (.92 ± .3 versus .7 ± .14, $P = NS$) (Zakowska-Dabrowska and Rybakowski 1973).

Finally, the invariable delay in cognitive improvement despite the lowering of serum lithium concentrations following treatment of acute lithium toxicity (DePaulo et al. 1982; El-Mallakh 1986a) is probably related to the slower time course in the reduction of intracellular lithium levels (see Chapter 3) (Pringuey et al. 1981).

Ionic Mechanism of Action

As intracellular lithium accumulates, it displaces sodium on a one-to-one basis (El-Mallakh 1990a; S. M. Friedman 1974; Haas et al. 1975). In lithium-treated rats, this is seen as a decrease in brain sodium (L. Baer et al. 1970b), and in humans, it can be detected as a decrease of the 24-hour exchangeable sodium (a measure of sodium entry into cells) and in residual sodium (Coppen et al. 1965).

Because lithium cannot appreciably substitute for sodium in sodium-calcium counterexchange, the reduction in available intracellular sodium reduces net calcium influx (Blaustein et al. 1980; Gill et al. 1984) or accelerates calcium efflux (Blaustein et al. 1980; Blaustein and Wiesmann 1970; Gill et al. 1984). Furthermore, chronic lithium treatment in animals (Meltzer et al. 1988) and in a small fraction of human bipolar patients (Hesketh et al. 1978) tends to increase Ca-ATPase pump activity, further decreasing intracellular calcium. The mechanism by which lithium increases Ca-ATPase activity is unknown but may involve an interaction with calmodulin (Meltzer 1993), an increase in the synthesis or expression of Ca-ATPase proteins (Meltzer et al. 1988), or both. The combined effect of these calcium changes would be to reduce the potency of the calcium signal postsynaptically (Dubovsky and Franks 1983) and the potency of the presynaptic calcium transient needed for neurotransmitter release (El-Mallakh 1990b; El-Mallakh and Jaziri 1990; El-Mallakh and Wyatt 1995).

Ionic substitution by lithium may take other forms. At therapeutic lithium concentrations, lithium can compete with magnesium at a low-affinity magnesium site on G proteins, thereby interfering with second-messenger transduction (see Chapter 5). At higher concentrations, lithium may interfere with a wide variety of magnesium-dependent enzymes (Gupta and Crollini 1974; Lazarus and Kitron 1974). Because the Na,K-ATPase and Ca-ATPase are both magnesium-dependent enzymes, inhibition of these systems may underlie the observed lithium toxicity-induced mania (El-Mallakh et al. 1987).

SUMMARY

Proper ionic control is essential for the proper functioning of all excitable tissue. Experimental evidence and plausible models suggest that significant alterations in ionic control are reliable mood-state markers in bipolar illness. Most significantly, there is an increase of both intracellular sodium and intracellular calcium concentration. Because of the key role of these ions in neuronal functioning, their dysregulation would be expected to result in significant neural dysfunction. By direct ionic displacement of sodium, and indirect displacement of calcium, lithium may contribute to the normalization of neuronal function.

Epilogue

Lithium is certainly the simplest psychopharmacological agent available, being a hydrated monocation in aqueous solutions (Schou 1957). Nonetheless, clear understanding of the mechanism by which it may produce its therapeutic and prophylactic effect in bipolar illness has been elusive despite more than four decades of clinical use and directed research (Cade 1949; Goodwin et al. 1969; Maggs 1963; Schou 1981). Understanding the mechanism of action of lithium would be invaluable in devising alternative (and perhaps safer) psychopharmacological agents, reducing the risk and consequences of lithium toxicity, and gaining valuable clues as to the pathophysiology of bipolar illness.

Lithium exerts a wide range of actions on a multitude of organs (especially the brain) (Ananth et al. 1987; El-Mallakh 1990b; Glue et al. 1987; Lewis 1982; Lippmann 1982; Mitchell and Mackenzie 1982) and produces a wide variety of cellular changes (Belmaker 1981; Berridge et al. 1982; Hokin-Neaverson and Jefferson 1989a; E. Klein et al. 1987; Vatal and Aiyar 1984). Although it is tempting to attempt to explain all lithium effects with one mechanism, it is much more likely that lithium exerts its actions via separate ionic and biochemical mechanisms. The ionic actions of lithium relate to its ability to displace and replace other biologically active inorganic cations (potassium, magnesium, calcium, and particularly sodium). The biochemical actions of lithium relate to its ability to interrupt or inhibit specific intracellular metabolic processes. The most important of these interruptions appears to be the inhibition of coupling or receptors with transducing G proteins (Avissar et al. 1988, 1991; Avissar and Schreiber 1989) and the inhibition of inositol phosphate breakdown with resultant disruption of the phosphatidylinositol cycle (Allison and Stewart 1971; Berridge et al. 1982; Hallcher and Sherman 1980; Ragan 1990). Unfortunately, there are as yet inadequate data examining the function of these systems in bipolar illness.

On the other hand, a multitude of studies have shown that Na,K-ATPase activity is a reliable mood-state marker in bipolar illness.

Specifically, Na,K-ATPase activity is decreased during acute phases of mood disturbance, with subsequent normalization accompanying mood recovery (El-Mallakh and Wyatt 1995). Several researchers believe that the sodium pump may play an important role in the pathogenesis of bipolar illness (El-Mallakh 1990a; El-Mallakh and Wyatt 1995; Naylor et al. 1980). An interaction between Na,K-ATPase and second messengers has been suggested (El-Mallakh and Li 1993) and opens the way to a greater understanding of the mechanism of lithium action.

Lithium treatment of bipolar patients (El-Mallakh and Wyatt 1995; Hokin-Neaverson and Jefferson 1989a) and of healthy human lymphocytes in vitro (Jenkins et al. 1991) is associated with an increase in Na,K-ATPase activity. The mechanism by which lithium accomplishes this is not clear but appears to be a result of an increase in the number of sodium pumps (Jenkins et al. 1991), an ability that may be reduced in bipolar subjects regardless of mood state (Naylor and Smith 1981).

Inositol, diacylglycerol (DAG), and protein kinase C all play a role in modulating the activity of the sodium pump. Inositol has long been known to be required for Na,K-ATPase to function properly (Charalampous 1971). More recently, work with experimental diabetes has helped clarify the relationship.

High glucose or galactose reduces the Na,K-ATPase of cells in tissue culture (Lee et al. 1989; Yorek et al. 1989, 1991a, 1991b) and peripheral nerves of diabetic rats (Das et al. 1976; Greene and Lattimer 1984; Hirata and Okada 1990; Kim et al. 1991a; Sonobe et al. 1991). The decreased sodium pump activity and consequent increase in intracellular sodium, particularly at the node of Ranvier (Brismar and Sima 1981; Greene et al. 1987), will block depolarization and produce the reductions in nerve conduction velocities seen in diabetic animals (Greene et al. 1975; Tomlinson and Mayer 1985) and humans (Troni et al. 1984). Sodium pump activity may be decreased secondary to a relative intracellular inositol deficiency resulting from decreased inositol uptake. Inositol uptake is sodium-dependent and can be competitively inhibited by glucose or galactose (Yorek et al. 1991a, 1991b). Diabetic patients will lose large amounts of inositol in the urine (Doughaday and Larner 1954), and the content of myoinositol in diabetic animal nerves may be decreased (Greene et al. 1987; Lu et al. 1990; Yorek and Dunlap 1991) or unchanged (Knudsen et al. 1989; Lee et al. 1989; Sonobe et al. 1991). However, myoinositol treatment or dietary supplementation will normalize Na,K-ATPase activity and nerve conduction velocities (Kim et al. 1991a; Tomlinson and Mayer 1985; Troni et al. 1984; Yorek et al. 1991a). The way in which myoinositol affects sodium pump activity is not clear. Whereas phosphatidylinositol (PI) may have sodium pump activating properties (Mandersloot et al. 1978; Roelofsen 1981), and there is good evidence that DAG and protein kinase C play significant roles, insulin will increase cellular DAG and protein kinase C activity but does not induce PI hydrolysis (D. R. Cooper et al. 1990). The elimination of insulin in the streptozocin-diabetic rat results in a decrease in the activity of cytosolic protein kinase C activity (Kim et al. 1991b) that parallels the drop in sodium pump activity in the sciatic nerve. Adding protein kinase C agonists in vitro (Vatal and Aiyar 1984) or ex vivo (Kim et al. 1991a) corrected Na,K-ATPase activity in diabetic tissue but had no effect on normal tissues. Myoinositol treatment or dietary supplementation also prevented the decrease in sodium pump activity (Kim et al. 1991a, 1991b; Vatal and Aiyar 1984). Myoinositol supplementation is believed to allow for replenishment of PI, PIP, and PIP_2 and renewed generations of DAG.

In other words, because states of myoinositol deficiency are associated with decreased sodium pump activity (Simmons and Winegard 1989), whereas states of myoinositol excess are generally without effect (Cohen et al. 1990; Greene et al. 1987), and because protein kinase C agonists increase sodium pump activity (Kim et al. 1991a; Vatal and Aiyar 1984), it appears unlikely that the observed reductions in Na,K-ATPase activity are secondary to a primary increase in phosphoinositide turnover. Conversely, it is proposed that a primary reduction in sodium pump activity results in a rise in intracellular sodium and intracellular calcium, as has been observed in acutely ill bipolar patients (Coppen et al. 1966; Dubovsky et al. 1989, 1991, 1992; D. M. Shaw 1966). These increases of intracellular sodium (Chandler and Crews 1990; Gusovsky et al. 1986, 1987) and calcium (Balduiri and Costa 1990; Brammer et al. 1988; Chandler and Crews 1990) may increase phosphoinositide hydrolysis, thereby generating the equivalent of a second-messenger signal in the absence of a first message (Figure E–1). Furthermore, because this artificial second message arose independently of a neurotransmitter signal, it may be resistant to a host of bypassed feedback controls, and it would be expected to last as long as the increased intracellular sodium and calcium concentrations persist. Lithium antagonizes this in several ways (Figure E–1). First, lithium prevents the formation of free myoinositol, thereby reducing PI, PIP, and PIP_2 regeneration (Berridge et al. 1982). Second, by depleting myoinositol, lithium slows the degradation of DAG (Busa and Gimlich 1989; Drummond and Raeburn 1984; Godfrey 1989; Kennedy et al. 1990; Watson et al. 1990), which through its effector, protein kinase C, can increase the activity of Na,K-ATPase in abnormal tissues (Kim et al. 1991a; Vatal and Aiyar 1984). Third, lithium may reduce intracellular calcium concentrations by accelerating Ca-ATPase activity (Meltzer 1990a, 1990b). Finally, lithium may directly reduce intracellular sodium concentrations by direct ionic replacement (El-Mallakh 1990a) (Figure E–1).

A variety of cellular or physiologic processes may produce reductions in sodium pump activity. For example, Naylor and Smith (1981) reported that cultured lymphocytes derived from bipolar patients are less capable than lymphocytes from healthy control subjects of increasing the number of sodium pump units in response to a stress that elevates intracellular sodium. This suggests that a defect in the regulation of Na,K-ATPase expression may underlie bipolar illness. Alternatively, dysregulation of the recently identified endogenous ouabain-like compounds (Hamlyn et al. 1991; Shaikh et al. 1991) may play a role in primary bipolar disorder (Christo and El-Mallakh 1993); on the other hand, because these compounds are apparently synthesized in the adrenal cortex, are quite lipophobic, and are present in relatively higher concentrations in the peripheral circulation (Hamlyn et al. 1991), they may play a role in secondary manias that occur in conjunction with pathologic processes that are associated with a breakdown of the blood-brain barrier.

Some of these speculations lend themselves to experimental validation. For example, as methods to quantify specific endogenous Na,K-ATPase inhibitors are perfected, it may be possible to

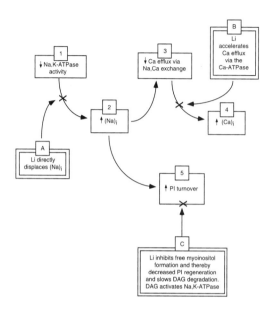

Figure E–1. A schematic proposal integrating the propounded mechanisms of lithium action.

1. Na,K-ATPase activity is decreased as a consequence of abnormal function or regulation in bipolar individuals.
2. This causes an increase in intracellular sodium.
3. The reduction in the sodium gradient slows the rate of calcium efflux via the sodium–calcium counterexchange pump.
4. This results in increased intracellular calcium.
5. The increase in intracellular sodium also activates phosphoinositide (PI) turnover via a process that requires extracellular calcium. The increase in PI turnover and intracellular calcium simulates a second message in the absence of a first message.

Lithium may counter these events at various sites.

A. Lithium could displace intracellular sodium on an ion-for-ion basis.
B. Lithium accelerates calcium efflux via the low-capacity calcium ATPase pump.
C. Lithium slows PI turnover by decreasing available myoinositol. The decrease of free myoinositol will also slow degradation of any DAG generated via hydolysis of PI. DAG, in turn, contributes to the correction of the original abnormality by increasing Na,K-ATPase activity.

measure these compounds directly in the peripheral circulation and cerebrospinal fluid of acutely ill and recovered bipolar patients. Furthermore, this question may be addressed in animal models of decreased neuronal pump activity (e.g., intracranially administered ouabain) or in cell cultures of lymphocytes derived from bipolar individuals and healthy control subjects. The model would predict that increases in intracellular sodium in these experimental systems would result in increased PI turnover and that chronic lithium treatment could prevent these changes.

These are exciting times. Answers to significant questions may be at hand. Work aimed at understanding the mechanism of lithium action will aid in unraveling the mystery of bipolar illness and help release millions of patients from the prison of unpredictable variability of bipolar illness.

References

Abdel-Latif AA, Brody J, Ranahi H: Studies on sodium-potassium adenosine triphosphatase of the nerve endings and appearance of electrical activity in developing rat brain. J Neurochem 14:1133–1141, 1967

Abdulla YH, Hamadah K: 3',5' Cyclic adenosine mono-phosphate in depression and mania (letter). Lancet 1:378, 1970

Abou-Saleh MT, Coppen A: Who responds to prophylactic lithium? J Affect Disord 10:115–125, 1986

Akagawa K, Watanabe M, Tsukada Y: Activity of erythrocyte Na,K-ATPase in manic patients. J Neurochem 35:258–260, 1980

Akiyam K, Vickroy TW, Watson M, et al: Muscarinic cholinergic ligand binding to intact mouse pituitary tumor cells coupling with two biochemical effectors: Adenylate cyclase and phosphatidyl inositol turnover. J Pharmacol Exp Ther 236:653–661, 1986

Albert KA, Helmer-Matyjck E, Nairn AC, et al: Calcium/phospholipid-dependent protein kinase (protein kinase C) phosphorylates and activates tyrosine hydroxylase. Proc Natl Acad Sci USA 81:7713–7717, 1984

Albrect J, Müller-Oerlinghausen B: Zur klinschen Bedeutung der intraerythozytären lithiumkonzentrtion: Ergebrisse einer katamnestischen Studie [Clinical relevance of lithium determination in RBC: Results of a catamnestic study]. Arzneim-Forsch 26:1145–1147, 1976.

Alexander DR, Deeb M, Bitar F, et al: Sodium-potassium, magnesium, and calcium ATPase activities in erythrocyte membranes from manic-depressive patients responding to lithium. Biol Psychiatry 21:997–1007, 1986

Alexander F, Martia J: Nephrotic syndrome associated with lithium therapy. Clin Nephrol 15:267–271, 1981

Alexander PE, van Kammen DP, Bunney WE Jr: Antipsychotic effects of lithium in schizophrenia. Am J Psychiatry 136:283–287, 1979

Allison JH, Blisner ME: Inhibition of the effect of lithium on brain inositol by atropine and scopolamine. Biochem Biophys Res Commun 68:1332–1338, 1976

Allison JH, Stewart MA: Reduced brain inositol in lithium-treated rats. Nature New Biol 233:267–268, 1971

Allison JH, Blisner ME, Holland WH, et al: Increased brain myoinositol-l-phosphate in lithium-treated rats. Biochem Biophys Res Commun 71:664–670, 1976

Almy GL, Taylor MA: Lithium retention in mania. Arch Gen Psychiatry 29:232–234, 1973

Amdisen A: Serum lithium estimations (letter). BMJ 2:240, 1973

American Psychiatric Association: Diagnostic and Statistical Manual of Mental Disorders, 4th Edition. Washington, DC, American Psychiatric Association, 1994

Amsterdam JD, Rybakowski J, Gottlieb J, et al: Kinetics of erythrocyte lithium-sodium countertransport in patients with affective illness before and during lithium therapy. J Affect Disord 14:75–81, 1988

Ananth J, Ghadirian AM, Engelsmann F: Lithium and memory: a review. Can J Psychiatry 32:312–316, 1987

Andersen PH, Geisler A: Lithium inhibition of forskolin-stimulated adenylate cyclase. Neuropsychobiology 12:1–3, 1984

Andersen PH, Klysner R, Geisler A: Forskolin-stimulated adenylate cyclase activity in rat cerebral cortex following chronic treatment with psychotropic drugs. Acta Pharmacol Toxicol 55:278–282, 1984

Anderson TW, Tiche WH, MacKay JS: Sudden death and ischemic heart disease: correlation with hardness of local water supply. N Engl J Med 280:805–807, 1969

Andriani G, Caselli G, Martelli G: Rilievi clinici ed elettroencefalografici durante il tatttamento con sali di litio in malati psichiatrici. Giornal Psichiatria Neuropatologia 86:273–328, 1958

Angst J, Dittrich A, Grof P: Course of endogenous affective psychoses and its modification by prophylactic administration of imipramine and lithium. Int Pharmacopsychiatry 2:1–11, 1969

Angst J, Weis P, Grof P, et al: Lithium prophylaxis in recurrent affective disorders. Br J Psychiatry 116:604–614, 1970.

Appleton WS, Davis JM: Practical Clinical Psychopharmacology, 2nd Edition. Baltimore, MD, Williams & Wilkins, 1980

Arminoff MJ, Marshall J: Treatment of Huntington's chorea with lithium carbonate: a double-blind trial. Lancet 1:107–109, 1974

Aronoff MS, Evens RG, Durell J: Effect of lithium salts on electrolyte metabolism. J Psychiatr Res 8:139–159, 1971

Åsberg M, Thorén P, Träskman L, et al: Serotonin depression: a biochemical subgroup within the affective disorders. Science 191:478–480, 1976

Ashby CD, Walsh DA: Characterization of the interaction of a protein inhibitor with adenosine 3'5'-monophosphate-dependent protein kinases, I: interaction with the catalytic subunit of the protein kinase. J Biol Chem 247:6637–6642, 1972

Atre-Vaidya N, Taylor MA: Effectiveness of lithium in schizophrenia: do we really have an answer? J Clin Psychiatry 50:170–173, 1989

Atterwill CK, Collins P: Studies on the ontogenesis of the different isoenzymes of NA⁺,K⁺-ATPase in rat brain in vivo and in vitro in relation to their regulation and cellular localization. Biochem Pharmacol 36:2679–2683, 1987

Avissar S, Schreiber G: Muscarinic receptor subclassification and G-proteins: significance for lithium action in affective disorders and for the treatment of the extrapyramidal side effects of neuroleptics. Biol Psychiatry 26:113–130, 1989

Avissar S, Schreiber G, Danon A, et al: Lithium inhibits adrenergic and cholinergic increases in GTP binding in rat cortex. Nature 331:440–442, 1988

Avissar S, Murphy DL, Schreiber G: Magnesium reversal of lithium inhibition of β-adrenergic and muscarinic receptor coupling to G proteins. Biochem Pharmacol 41:171–175, 1991

Baastrup PC: The use of lithium in manic-depressive psychosis. Compr Psychiatry 5:396–408, 1964

Baastrup PC, Schou M: Lithium as a prophylactic agent: its effect against recurrent depression and manic-depressive psychosis. Arch Gen Psychiatry 16:162–172, 1967

Baastrup PC, Poulsen JC, Schou M, et al: Prophylactic lithium: double-blind discontinuation in manic-depressive and recurrent depressive disorders. Lancet 2:326–330, 1970

Baastrup PC, Hollnagel P, Sorensen R, et al: Adverse reactions in treatment with lithium carbonate and haloperidol. JAMA 236:2645–2646, 1976

Baer L, Burell J, Bunney WE Jr, et al : Sodium balance and distribution in lithium carbonate therapy. Arch Gen Psychiatry 22:40–44, 1970a

Baer L, Kassir S, Fieve R: Lithium-induced changes in electrolyte balance and tissue electrolyte concentrations. Psychopharmacologia 17:216–224, 1970b

Baer RA, Paul M: Nephrotic syndrome and renal failure secondary to lithium carbonate therapy. Can Med Assoc J 132:735–737, 1985

Baker PF: Transport and metabolism of calcium ions in nerve. Prog Biophys Mol Biol 24:177–223, 1972

Baker PF, Blaustein MP, Hodgkin AL: The influence of calcium on sodium efflux in squid axons. J Physiol (Lond) 1969;200:431–458

Baldessarini RJ: Chemotherapy in Psychiatry, Principles and Practice. Cambridge, MA, Harvard University Press, 1985

Baldessarini RJ, Lipinski JF: Lithium salts: 1970–1975. Ann Intern Med 83:527–533, 1975

Baldessarini RJ, Stephens JH: Lithium carbonate for affective disorders: clinical pharmacology and toxicology. Arch Gen Psychiatry 22:72–77, 1970

Balduiri W, Costa LG: Characterization of ouabain-induced phospho-inositide hydrolysis in brain slices in neonatal rat. Neurochem Res 15:1023–1029, 1990

Ball JH, Kaminsky NI, Hardman JG, et al: Effects of catecholamines and adrenergic-blocking agents on plasma and urinary cyclic nucleotides in man. J Clin Invest 51:2124–2129, 1972

Banks RE, Aiton JF, Cramb G, et al: Incorporation of inositol into the phosphinositides of lymphoblastoid cell lines established from bipolar manic-depressive patients. J Affect Disord 19:1–8, 1990

Baraban JM, Snyder SH, Alger BE: Protein kinase C regulates ionic conductances in hippocampal pyramidal neurons: electrophysiological effects of phorbol esters. Proc Natl Acad Sci USA 82:2538–2542, 1985

Baraban JM, Worley PF, Snyder SH: Second messenger systems and psychoactive drug action: focus on the phosphoinositide system and lithium. Am J Psychiatry 146:1251–1260, 1989

Barkai AI: Myoinositol turnover in the intact rat brain: increased production after d-amphetamine. J Neurochem 36:1485–1491, 1981

Baron M, Gershon ES, Rudy V, et al: Lithium carbonate response in depression: prediction by unipolar/bipolar illness, average-evoked response, catechol-O-methyl transferase, and family history. Arch Gen Psychiatry 32:1107–1111, 1975

Barrett AJ, Hugh-Jones K, Newton K, et al: Lithium therapy in aplastic anaemia (letter). Lancet 1:202, 1977

Barrett AJ, Griscelli C, Buriot D, et al: Lithium therapy in congenital neutropenia: correlation between clinical response and in vitro studies. Pediatr Res 13:429–431, 1979

Battle DC, von Riotte AB, Gaviria M, et al: Amelioration of polyuria by amelioride in patients receiving long-term lithium therapy. N Engl J Med 312:408–414, 1985

Beardsley RS, Gardocki GJ, Larson DB, et al: Prescribing of psychotropic medication by primary care physicians and psychiatrists. Arch Gen Psychiatry 45:1117–1119, 1988

Belling G: Lithium-behandling på et sindssygehospital. Ugeskr Laeger 121:1193–1195, 1959

Belmaker RH: Receptors, adenylate cyclase, depression and lithium. Biol Psychiatry 16:333–350, 1981

Belmaker RH, Schreiber-Avissar S, Schreiber G, et al: Does the effect of lithium on G-proteins have behavioral correlates? in Lithium and Cell Physiology. Edited by Bach RO, Gallichio VS. New York, Springer-Verlag, 1990a, pp 94–101

Belmaker, RH, Livne A, Agam G, et al: Role of inositol-1-phosphatase inhibition in the mechanism of action of lithium. Pharmacol Toxicol 60(suppl 3):76–83, 1990b

Bennett CF, Balcauk JM, Varrichio A, et al: Molecular cloning and complete sequence of form-I phosphoinositide-specific phospholipase C. Nature 334:268–270, 1988

Berl S, Clarke DD: Lithium and amino acid metabolism, in Lithium Research and Therapy. Edited by Johnson FN. London, Academic Press, 1975, pp 425–441

Berrebi-Bertrand I, Maixent J-M, Christe G, et al: Two active NA^+/K^+-ATPases of high affinity for ouabain in adult rat brain membranes. Biochim Biophys Acta 1021:148–156, 1990

Berrettini WH, Nurnberger JI Jr, Hare TA, et al: Reduced plasma and CSF β-aminobutyric acid in affective illness. Biol Psychiatry 18:185–194, 1983

Berridge MJ: Inositol triphosphate and diacylglycerol as second messengers. Biochem J 220:345–360, 1984

Berridge MJ: Inositol triphosphate and diacylglycerol: two interacting second messengers. Annu Rev Biochem 56:159–193, 1987

Berridge MJ, Downes CP, Hanley MR: Lithium amplifies agonist-dependent phosphatidylinositol responses in brain and salivary glands. Biochem J 206:587–595, 1982

Billah MM, Anthes JC: The regulation and cellular functions of phosphatidylcholine hydrolysis. Biochem J 269:281–291, 1990

Birnbaum J, Klandorf H, Giuliano A, et al: Lithium stimulates the release of human parathyroid hormone in vitro. J Clin Endocrinol Metab 66:1187–1191, 1988

Blackwell B: Prophylactic lithium: science or science fiction? Am Heart J 83:139–141, 1972

Blackwell B, Shepherd M: Prophylactic lithium: another therapeutic myth? an examination of the evidence to date. Lancet 1:968–971, 1968

Blaustein MP: The interrelationship between sodium and calcium fluxes across cell membranes. Rev Physiol Biochem Pharmacol 70:33–82, 1974

Blaustein MP: Calcium transport and buffering in neurons. Trend Neuro Sci 11:438–442, 1988

Blaustein MP, Wiesmann WP: Effect of sodium ions on calcium movements in isolated synaptic terminals. Proc Natl Acad Sci USA 66:664–671, 1970

Blaustein MP, Russell JM, DeWeer P: Calcium efflux from internally dialyzed squid axons: the influence of external and internal cations. J Supramol Struct 2:558–581, 1974

Blaustein MP, Ratzluff RW, Schwitzer ES: Control of intracellular calcium in presynaptic nerve terminals. Fed Proc 39:2790–2795, 1980

Blinder MG: Some observations on the use of lithium carbonate. Int J Neurol 4:26–27, 1968

Bliss EL, Ailion J: The effect of lithium upon brain neuroamines. Brain Res 24:305–310, 1970

Boer WH, Joles JA, Koomans HA, et al: Decreased lithium clearance due to distal tubular lithium reabsorption in sodium-depleted dogs. Renal Physiol (Basel) 10:65–68, 1987

Bond PA, Jenner FA, Sampson CA: Daily variations of the urine content of MHPG in two manic-depressive patients. Psychol Med 2:81–85, 1972

Bowers MB Jr, Heninger GR, Gerbode F: Cerebrospinal fluid 5-hydroxyindoleacetic acid and homovanillic acid in psychiatric patients. Int J Neuropharmacol 8:255–259, 1969

Brammer MJ, Hajimohammadreza I, Sawdiwal S, et al: Is inositol bisphosphate the product of A23187 and carbachol-mediated phosphoinositide breakdown in synaptosomes? J Neurochem 51:414–421, 1988

Brandt DR, Ross EM: Catecholamine-stimulated GTPase cycle: multiple sites of regulation by β-adrenergic receptor and Mg^{2+} studied in reconstituted receptor-Gs vesicles. J Biol Chem 261:1656–1664, 1986

Brewenton TD: Lithium counteracts carbamazepine-induced leukopenia while increasing its therapeutic effect. Biol Psychiatry 21:677–685, 1986

Brismar T, Sima AAF: Changes in nodal function in nerve fibers of the spontaneously diabetic BB-Sistar rat: potential clamp analysis. Acta Physiol Scand 113:499–506, 1981

Brodsky JL, Guidotti G: Sodium affinity of brain Na^+, K^+-ATPase is dependent on isoenzymes and environment of the pnm. Am J Physiol (Cell Physiol 27): C803–C811, 1990

Brooks SC, Lessin BE: Treatment of resistant lithium-induced nephrogenic diabetes insipidus and schizoaffective psychosis with carbamazepine. Am J Psychiatry 140:1077–1078, 1983

Brown EM: Lithium induces abnormal calcium-regulated PTH release in dispersed bovine parathyroid cells. J Clin Endocrinol Metab 52:1046–1048, 1981

Brown RP, Ingber PS, Tross S: Pemoline and lithium in a patient with attention deficit disorder. J Clin Psychiatry 44:146–148, 1983

Brown WT: Side effects of lithium therapy and their treatment. Can Psychiatr Assoc J 21:13–21, 1976

Bruzzone R: The molecular basis of enzyme secretion. Gastroenterol 99:1157–1176, 1990

Bunney WE Jr, Davis J: Norepinephrine in depressive reactions. Arch Gen Psychiatry 13:483–494, 1965

Bunney WE Jr, Goodwin FK, Davis JM, et al: A behavioral-biochemical study of lithium treatment. Am J Psychiatry 125:499–512, 1968

Burrows GD, Davies R, Kincaid-Smith P: Unique tubular lesion after lithium (letter). Lancet 1:1310, 1978

Busa WB, Gimlich RL: Lithium-induced teratogenesis in frog embryos prevented by a polyphosphoinositide cycle, intermediate or a diacylglycerol analog. Dev Biol 132:315–324, 1989

Cade JFJ: Lithium salts in the treatment of psychotic excitement. Med J Aust 36:349–352, 1949

Calabrese JR, Delucchi GA: Spectrum of efficacy of valproate in 55 patients with rapid-cycling bipolar disorder. Am J Psychiatry 147:431–434, 1990

Calabrese JR, Gulledge AD, Hahn K, et al: Autoimmune thyroiditis in manic-depressive patients treated with lithium. Am J Psychiatry 142:1318–1321, 1985

Calabrese JR, Markovitz PJ, Kimmel SE, et al: Spectrum of efficacy of valproate in 78 rapid-cycling bipolar patients. J Clin Psychopharmacol 12:535–565, 1992

Campbell M, Spencer EK: Psychopharmacology in child and adolescent psychiatry: a review of the past five years. J Am Acad Child Adolesc Psychiatry 27:269–279, 1988

Carafoli E, Crompton M: The regulation of intracellular calcium by mitochondria. Ann NY Acad Sci 307:269–284, 1978

Carafoli E, Longoni S: The plasma membrane in the control of the signaling function of calcium, in Cell Calcium and the Control of Membrane Transport. Edited by Mandel LJ, Eaton DC. New York, The Rockefeller University Press, 1987, pp 21–29

Carlson GA, Kashani JH: Manic symptoms in a non-referred adolescent population. J Affect Disord 15:219–226, 1988

Carman JS, Bigelow LB, Wyatt RJ: Lithium combined with neuroleptics in chronic schizophrenic and schizoaffective patients. J Clin Psychiatry 42:124–128, 1981

Casebolt TL, Jope RS: Chronic lithium treatment reduces norepinephrine-stimulated inositol phospholipid hydrolysis in rat cortex. Eur J Pharmacol 140: 245–246, 1987

Casebolt TL, Jope RS: Effects of chronic lithium treatment on protein kinase C and cyclic AMP-dependent protein phosphorylation. Biol Psychiatry 29:233–243, 1991

Casper RC, Pandey G, Gosenfeld L, et al: Intracellular lithium and clinical response. Lancet 2:418–419, 1976

Cassel D, Selinger Z: Mechanism of adenylate cyclase activation through the beta-adrenergic receptor: catecholamine-induced displacement of bound GDP by DTP. Proc Natl Acad Sci USA 75:4155–4159, 1978

Castellucci VF, Kandel ER, Schwartz JH, et al: Intracellular injection of the catalytic subunit of cyclic AMP-dependent protein kinase stimulates facilitation of transmitter release underlying behavioral sensitization in aplasia. Proc Natl Acad Sci USA 77:7492–7496, 1980

Cazzullo CL, Smeraldi E, Sacchetti E, et al: Intracellular lithium concentration and clinical response. Br J Psychiatry 126:298–300, 1975

Cervi-Skinner SJ: Lithium carbonate induced hypercalcemia. West J Med 127:527–528, 1977

Chandler LJ, Crews FT: Calcium-versus G protein-mediated phosphoinositide hydrolysis in rat cerebral cortical synaptoneurosomes. J Neurochem 55:1022–1030, 1990

Chang Y-C, Li H-N, Deng H-C: Subclinical lithium neurotoxicity: correlation of neural conduction abnormalities and serum lithium level in manic-depressive patients with lithium treatment. Acta Neurol Scand 82:82–86, 1990

Charalampous FC: Metabolic functions of myoinositol, VIII: role of inositol in Na^+-K^+ transport and in Na^+- and K^+-activated adenosine triphosphatase of KB cells. J Biol Chem 246:455–460, 1971

Choi SJ, Taylor MA, Abrams R: Depression, ECT, and erythrocyte adenosinetriphosphatase activity. Biol Psychiatry 12:75–81, 1977

Chouinard G: The use of benzodiazepines in the treatment of manic-depressive illness. J Clin Psychiatry 49(suppl 11):15–19, 1988

Chouinard G, Steiner W: Remoxipride in the treatment of acute mania. Biol Psychiatry 21:1429–1433, 1986

Christiansen C, Baastrup PC, Transbol I: Development of "primary" hyperparathyroidism during lithium therapy: longitudinal study. Neuropsychobiology 6:280–283, 1980

Christo PJ, El-Mallakh RS: Possible role of endogenous ouabain-like compounds in the pathophysiology of bipolar illness. Med Hyphotheses 41:378–383, 1993

Civan MM, Shporer M: Physical state of cell sodium, in Cellular and Molecular Biology of Sodium Transport. Current Topics in Membrane Transport Vol 1. Edited by Hoffman JF, Giebisch G, Schultz SG. San Diego, CA, Academic Press 1989, pp 1–19

Cochran SD: Compliance with lithium regimens in the outpatient treatment of bipolar affective disorders. J Compliance Health Care 1:153–170, 1986

Cocoran AC, Taylor RD, Page IH: Lithium poisoning from the use of salt substitutes. JAMA 139:685–688, 1949

Coffey CE, Ross DR, Ferren EL, et al: Treatment of the "on-off" phenomenon in Parkinsonism with lithium carbonate. Ann Neurol 12:375–379, 1982

Cohen RA, MacGregor LC, Spokes KC, et al: Effect of myoinositol on Renal Na, K-ATPase in experimental diabetes. Metabolism 39:1026–1032, 1990

Collado S, Charron D, Degos L: Double-blind, placebo-controlled lithium treatment in chemotherapy-induced aplasia for AML: reduced antibiotic requirement. Med Oncol Tumor Pharmacother 5:103–105, 1988

Cooper DMF, Bier-Laning AM, Halford MK, et al: Dopamine acting through D_2 receptors inhibits rat striatal adenylate cyclase by a GTP-dependent process. Mol Pharmacol 29:113–119, 1986

Cooper DR, Hernandez H, Kuo JY, et al: Insulin increases the synthesis of phospholipid and diacylglycerol and protein kinase C activity in rat hepatocytes. Arch Biochem Biophys 276:486–494, 1990

Cooper TB, Bergner PEE, Simpson GM: The 24-hour serum lithium level as a prognosticator of dosage requirement. Am J Psychiatry 130:601–603, 1973

Coppen A, Shaw DM: Mineral metabolism in melancholia. Br Med J 2:1439–1444, 1963

Coppen A, Malleson A, Shaw DM: Effects of lithium carbonate on electrolyte distribution in man. Lancet 2:682–683, 1965

Coppen A, Shaw DM, Malleson A, et al: Mineral metabolism in mania. Brit J Med 1:71–75, 1966

Coppen A, Noguera R, Baily J, et al: Prophylactic lithium in affective disorders: controlled trial. Lancet 2:275–279, 1971

Coppen A, Prange AJ Jr, Whybrow PC, et al: Abnormalities of indoleamines in affective disorders. Arch Gen Psychiatry 26:474–478, 1972

Coppen A, Swade C, Wood K: Platelet 5-hydroxytryptamine accumulation in depressive illness. Clin Chim Acta 87:165–168, 1978

Cordess C: "Rebound" mania after lithium withdrawal? (letter) Br J Psychiatry 141:431, 1982

Corrodi H, Fuxe K, Schou M: The effect of prolonged lithium administration on cerebral monoamine neurons in the rat. Life Sci 8:643–651, 1969

Corthesy-Theulaz I, Merillat A-M, Honegger P, et al: Na^+-K^+-ATPase gene expression during in vivo development of rat fetal forebrain. Am J Physiol 258:C1062–C1069, 1990

Costa MRC, Catterall WA: Cyclic AMP-dependent phosphorylation of the α subunit of the sodium channel in synaptic nerve ending particles. J Biol Chem 259:8210–8218, 1984a

Costa MRC, Catterall WA: Phosphorylation in the α subunit of the sodium channel by protein kinase C. Cell Mol Neurobiol 4:291–297, 1984b

Costa MRC, Casnellie JE, Catterall WA: Selective phosphorylation of the α subunit of the sodium channel by cAMP-dependent protein kinase. J Biol Chem 257:7918–7921, 1982

Cubitt AB, Geras-Raaka E, Gershengorn MC: Thyrotropin-releasing hormone receptor occupancy determines the fraction of the responsive pool of inositol lipids hydrolyzed in rat pituitary tumour cells. Biochem J 271(2):331–336, 1990

Cummings JL, Benson DF: The nucleus basalis of Meynert in dementia: a review and reconsideration. Alzheimer Dis Assoc Disord 1:128–145, 1987

Cummings MA, Cummings KL, Haviland MG: Use of potassium to treat lithium's side effects (letter). Am J Psychiatry 145:895, 1988

Cundall RL, Brooks PW, Murray LG: A controlled evaluation of lithium prophylaxis in affective disorders. Psychol Med 2:308–311, 1972

Dagher G, Gay C, Brossard M, et al: Lithium, sodium, and potassium transport in erythrocytes of manic-depressive patients. Acta Psychiatr Scand 69:24–36, 1984

Dalen P: Lithium therapy in Huntington's chorea and tardive dyskinesia. Lancet 1:107–108, 1973

Daniell LC, Harris RA: Ethanol and inositol 1,4,5-triphosphate release calcium from separate stores in brain microsomes. J Pharmacol Exp Ther 250:875–881, 1989

Das PK, Bray GM, Aguayo AJ, et al: Diminished ouabain-sensitive sodium potassium ATPase activity in sciatic nerves of rats with streptozotocin induced diabetes. Exp Neurol 53:285–288, 1976

Davis JM: Overview: maintenance therapy in psychiatry, II: affective disorders. Am J Psychiatry 133:1–13, 1976

Davis KL, Berger PA, Hollister LE, et al: Physostigmine in mania. Arch Gen Psychiatry 35:119–122, 1978

Decina P, Oliver JA, Sciacca RR, et al: Effect of lithium therapy on glomerular filtration rate. Am J Psychiatry 140:1065–1067, 1983

de la Fuente J-R, Morse RM, Niven RG, et al: A controlled study of lithium carbonate in the treatment of alcoholism. Mayo Clin Proc 64:177–180, 1989

DeLong GR, Aldershof AL: Long-term experience with lithium treatment in childhood: correlation with clinical diagnosis. J Am Acad Child Adolesc Psychiatry 26:389–394, 1987

Delva NJ, Letemerdia FJJ: Lithium treatment in schizophrenia and schizoaffective disorders. Br J Psychiatry 141:387–400, 1982

Demers RG, Heninger GR: Electrocardiographic T-wave changes during lithium carbonate. JAMA 218:381–386, 1971

dé Montigny C, Grunberg F, Mayer A, et al: Lithium induces rapid relief of depression in tricyclic antidepressant drug non-responders. Br J Psychiatry 138:252–256, 1981 dé Montigny C, Couenoyer G, Morissette R, et al: Lithium carbonate addition in tricyclic antidepressant-resistant unipolar depression: correlations with the neurobiologic actions of tricyclic antidepressant drugs and lithium ion on the serotonin system. Arch Gen Psychiatry 40:1327–1334, 1983

dé Montigny C, Elie R, Caillé G: Rapid response to the addition of lithium in ipridole-resistant unipolar depression: a pilot study. Am J Psychiatry 142:220–223, 1985

Dempsey M, Dunner DL, Fieve RR, et al: Treatment of excessive weight gain in patients taking lithium. Am J Psychiatry 133:1082–1084, 1976

DePaulo JR Jr, Folstein MF, Correa EL: The course of delirium due to lithium intoxication. J Clin Psychiatry 43:447–449, 1982

Depner TA: Nephrotic syndrome secondary to lithium therapy. Nephron 30:286–271, 1982

Dias H, Hochen AG: Oliguric renal failure complicating lithium carbonate therapy. Nephron 20:246–249, 1972

Dilsaver SC: Lithium's effects on muscarinic receptor binding parameters: a relationship to therapeutic efficacy? Biol Psychiatry 19:1551–1565, 1984

Dilsaver SC: Cholinergic mechanisms in depression. Brain Res 396:285–316, 1986

Donaldson JO, Hale MS, Klau M: A case of reversible pure-work deafness during lithium toxicity. Am J Psychiatry 138:242–243, 1981

Dorus E, Cox NJ, Gibbons RD, et al: Lithium of a major gene locus. Arch Gen Psychiatry 40:545–552, 1983

Doughaday WH, Larner J: The renal excretion of inositol in normal and diabetic human beings. J Clin Invest 33:326–332, 1954

Dousa T, Hechter O: The effect of NaCl and LiCl on vasopressin-sensitive adenyl cyclase. Life Sci 9:765–770, 1970

Downes CP: Receptor-stimulated inositol phospholipid metabolism in the central nervous system. Cell Calcium 3:413–428, 1982

Drummond AH, Raeburn CA: The interaction of lithium with thyrotropin releasing hormone-stimulated lipid metabolism in GH_3 pituitary tumor cells. Biochem J 224:129–136, 1984

Dubovsky SL, Franks RD: Intracellular calcium ions in affective disorders: a review and an hypothesis. Biol Psychiatry 18:781–797, 1983

Dubovsky SL, Franks RD, Allen S: Verapamil: a new antimanic drug with potential interactions with lithium. J Clin Psychiatry 48:371–372, 1987

Dubovsky SL, Christiano J, Daniell LC, et al: Increased platelet intracellular calcium concentration in patients with bipolar affective disorders. Arch Gen Psychiatry 46:632–638, 1989

Dubovsky SL, Lee C, Christiano J, et al: Elevated platelet intracellular calcium concentration in bipolar depression. Biol Psychiatry 29:441–450, 1991

Dubovsky SL, Murphy J, Thomas M, et al: Abnormal intracellular calcium ion concentration in platelets and lymphocytes of bipolar patients. Am J Psychiatry 149:118–120, 1992

Dunner DL, Fieve RR: Clinical factors in lithium carbonate prophylaxis failure. Arch Gen Psychiatry 30:229–233, 1974

Dvoredsky AE, Stewart MA: Hyperactivity followed by manic-depressive disorder: two case reports. J Clin Psychiatry 42:212–214, 1981

Dyson WL, Mendels J: Lithium and depression. Curr Ther Res Clin Exp 10:601–608, 1968

Ebstein R, Belmaker R, Grunhaus L, et al: Lithium inhibition of adrenaline-stimulated adenylate cyclase in humans. Nature 259:411–413, 1976

Ebstein RP, Hermoni M, Belmaker RH: The effect of lithium on noradrenaline-induced cyclic AMP accumulation in rat brain; inhibition after chronic treatment and absence of supersensitivity. J Pharmacol Exp Ther 213:161–167, 1980

Ehrlich BE, Diamond JM: Lithium fluxes in human erythrocytes. Am J Physiol 237(6):C102–C110, 1979

Ehrlich BE, Diamond JM, Kaye W, et al: Lithium transport in erythrocytes from a pair of twins with manic disorder. Am J Psychiatry 136:1477–1478, 1979

Ehrlich BE, Diamond JM, Gosenfeld L: Lithium-induced changes in sodium-lithium countertransport. Biochem Pharmacol 30:2539–2543, 1981

Eisner DA, Lederer WJ: Characterization of the electrogenic sodium pump in cardiac Purkinje fibers. Journal of Psychobiology 303:441–474, 1980

Eliasen P, Andersen M: Sinoatrial block during lithium treatment. Eur J Cardiol 3:97–98, 1975

Ellis J, Lenox RH: Chronic lithium treatment prevents atropine-induced supersensitivity of the muscarinic phosphoinositide response in rat hippocampus. Biol Psychiatry 28:609–619, 1990

Ellis J, Lenox RH: Receptor coupling to G proteins: interactions not affected by lithium. Lithium 2:141–147, 1991

El-Mallakh RS: The Na,K-ATPase hypothesis for manic-depression, I: general considerations. Med Hypotheses 12:253–268, 1983a

El-Mallakh RS: The Na,K-ATPase hypothesis for manic-depression, II: the mechanism of action of lithium. Med Hypotheses 12:269–282, 1983b

El-Mallakh RS: Treatment of acute lithium toxicity. Vet Hum Toxicol 26:31–35, 1984

El-Mallakh RS: Acute lithium neurotoxicity. Psychiatr Dev 4:311–328, 1986a

El-Mallakh RS: Hypertension and diabetes in obesity: a review and new ideas on the contributing role of ions. Med Hypotheses 19:47–55, 1986b

El-Mallakh RS: Complications of concurrent lithium and electroconvulsive therapy: a review of clinical material and theoretical considerations. Biol Psychiatry 23:595–601, 1988

El-Mallakh RS: The ionic mechanism of lithium action. Lithium 1:87–92, 1990a

El-Mallakh RS: Lithium. Conn Med 54:115–126, 1990b

El-Mallakh RS: Preventing bipolar relapse while avoiding lithium toxicity: the role of the lithium ratio and intradrythrocyte lithium concentration determination. Lithium 5:17–22, 1994

El-Mallakh RS, Jaziri WA: Calcium channel blockers in affective illness: role of sodium-calcium exchange. J Clin Psychopharmacol 10:203–206, 1990

El-Mallakh RS, Lee RH: Seizures and transient cognitive deterioration as sequelae of acute lithium intoxication. Vet Hum Toxicol 29:143–145, 1987

El-Mallakh RS, Li R: Is the Na,K-ATPase the link between phosphoinositide metabolism and bipolar disorder? J Neuropsychiatry Clin Neurosci 5:361–368, 1993

El-Mallakh RS, Wyatt RJ: The Na,K-ATPase hypothesis for bipolar illness. Biol Psychiatry 37:235–244, 1995

El-Mallakh RS, Kantesaria AN, Chaikovsky LI: Lithium toxicity presenting as mania. Drug Intell Clin Pharm 21:979–981, 1987

El-Mallakh RS, Kirch DG, Shelton R, et al: The nucleus basalis of Meynert, senile plaques, and intellectual impairment in schizophrenia. J Neuropsychiatry Clin Neurosci 3:383–386, 1991

El-Mallakh RS, Barrett JL, Wyatt RJ: The Na,K-ATPase hypothesis for bipolar disorder: implications of normal development. Journal of Child and Adolescent Psychopharmacology 3:37–52, 1993

Emerson CH, Dyson WL, Utinger RD: Serum thyrotropin and thyroxine concentrations in patients receiving lithium carbonate. J Clin Endocrinol Metab 36:338–346, 1973

Epstein R, Grant L, Herjanic M, et al: Urinary excretion of lithium in mania (letter). JAMA 192:149, 1965

Erwin CW, Gerber CJ, Morrison SD, et al: Lithium carbonate and convulsive disorders. Arch Gen Psychiatry 28:646–648, 1973

Escobar JI, Skoutakis VA: Management of lithium over-dosages. Clinical Toxicology Consultant 1:102–118, 1979

Ezrin-Waters C, Resch L: The nucleus basalis of Meynert. Can J Neurol Sci 13:8–14, 1986

Faedda GL, Tondo L, Baldessarini RJ, et al: Outcome after rapid vs. gradual discontinuation of lithium treatment in bipolar disorders. Arch Gen Psychiatry 50:448–455, 1993

Fawcett J, Clark DC, Aagesen CA, et al: A double-blind, placebo-controlled trial of lithium carbonate therapy for alcoholism. Arch Gen Psychiatry 44:248–256, 1987

Feighner JP, Aden GC, Fabre LF, et al: Comparison of alprazolam, imipramine, and placebo in the treatment of major depression. JAMA 249:3057–3064, 1983

Feinberg M, Steiner M, Carrol BJ: Effects of long-term lithium treatment on serum calcium, magnesium and calcitonin. Psychopharmacol Bull 11:81–84, 1979

Feinstein SF, Wolpert EA: Juvenile manic-depressive illness: clinical and therapeutic considerations. J Am Acad Child Adolesc Psychiatry 12:123–136, 1973

Fieve RR, Kumbaraci T, Dunner DL: Lithium prophylaxis of depression in bipolar I, bipolar II, and unipolar patients. Am J Psychiatry 133:925–930, 1976

Fink M: Electroencephalogram, the mental state, and psychoactive drugs. Pharmacol Physicians 3:1, 1969

Fisher SK, Agranoff BW: Receptor activation and inositol lipid hydrolysis in neural tissues. J Neurochem 48:999–1017, 1987

Fisher SK, Heacock AM, Agranoff BW: Inositol lipids and signal transduction in the nervous system: an update. J Neurochem 58:18–38, 1991

Flemenbaum A, Weddige R, Miller J Jr: Lithium erythrocyte/plasma ratio as a predictor of response. Am J Psychiatry 135:336–338, 1978

Fleming JW, Watanabe AM: Muscarinic cholinergic-receptor stimulation of specific GTP hydrolysis related to adenylate cyclase activity in canine cardiac sarcolemma. Circ Res 64:340–350, 1988

Fontaine R, Ontiveros A, Elie R, et al: Lithium carbonate augmentation of desipramine and fluoxetine in refractory depression. Biol Psychiatry 29:946–948, 1991

Forn J, Valdecasas FG: Effects of lithium on brain adenyl cyclase activity. Biochem Pharmacol 20:2773–2779, 1971

Forrest JN Jr, Cohen AD, Torretti J, et al: On the mechanism of lithium-induced diabetes insipidus in man and the rat. J Clin Invest 53:1115–1123, 1974

Forrest JN Jr, Cox M, Hong C, et al: Superiority of demeclocycline over lithium in the treatment of chronic syndrome of inappropriate secretion of antidiuretic hormone. N Engl J Med 298:173–177, 1978

Fowler NO, McCall D, Chou TC, et al: Electrocardiographic changes and cardiac arrhythmias in patients receiving psychotropic drugs. Am J Cardiol 37:223–230, 1976

Frazer A, Secunda SK, Mendels J: A method for the determination of sodium, potassium, magnesium, and lithium concentrations in erythrocytes. Clin Chim Acta 36:499–509, 1972

Frazer A, Mendels J, Secunda SK, et al: The prediction of brain lithium concentrations from plasma or erythrocyte measures. J Psychiatr Res 10:1–7, 1973

Frazer A, Mendels J, Brunswick D: Transfer of lithium ions across the erythrocyte membrane. Commun Psychopharmacol 1:1255–1270, 1977

Friedman E, Gershon S: Effect of lithium on brain dopamine. Nature 243:520–521, 1973

Friedman SM: Lithium substitution and the distribution of sodium in the rat tail artery. Circ Res 34:168–175, 1974

Fukunaga K, Rich DP, Soderling TR: Generation of the Ca^{2+}-independent form of calcium/calmodulin-dependent protein kinase II in cerebellar granule cells. J Biol Chem 264:21830–21836, 1989

Gallager DW, Pert A, Bunney WE Jr: Haloperidol-induced presynaptic dopamine supersensitivity is blocked by chronic lithium. Nature 273:309–312, 1978

Gandhi CR, Ross DH: Inositol 1,4,5-triphosphate induced mobilization of Ca^{2+} from rat brain synaptosomes. Neurochem Res 12:67–72, 1987

Garson OM, Latimer NZ, Chiu E, et al: Chromosome studies of patients on long-term lithium therapy for psychiatric disorders. Med J Aust 2:37–39, 1981

Garver DL, Hirschowitz J, Fleishman R, et al: Lithium response and psychoses: a double-blind, placebo-controlled study. Psychiatry Res 12:57–68, 1984

Gelenberg AJ: Lithium efficacy and adverse effects. J Clin Psychiatry 49(suppl 11):8–9, 1988

Gelenberg AJ, Kane JM, Keller MB, et al: Comparison of standard and low serum levels of lithium for maintenance treatment of bipolar disorder. N Engl J Med 321:1489–1493, 1989

Gengo F, Timko J, D'Antonio J, et al: The utility of a single-point dosing protocol for predictive method. J Clin Psychiatry 130:601–603, 1973

Gerlach J, Thorsen K, Munkvad I: Effect of lithium on neuroleptic-induced tardive dyskinesia compared with placebo in a double-blind cross-over trial. Pharmakopsychiatrie 8:51–56, 1975

Gerner RH, Post RM, Bunney WE Jr: A dopaminergic mechanism in mania. Am J Psychiatry 133:1177–1180, 1976

Gershon S, Trautner EM: The treatment of shock-dependency by pharmacological agents. Med J Aust 43:783–787, 1956

Gershon S, Yuwiler A: Lithium ion: a specific psychopharmacological approach to the treatment of mania. J Neuropsychiatry Clin Neurosci 1:229–241, 1960

Gill DC, Chueh S-H, Whitlow CL: Functional importance of the synaptic plasma membrane calcium pump and sodium-calcium exchange. J Biol Chem 259:10807–10813, 1984

Gilman AG: G-proteins: transducers of receptor-generated signals. Annu Rev Biochem 56:615–649, 1987

Girke W, Krebs FA, Müller-Oerlinghausen B: Effects of lithium on electromyographic recording in man. Int Pharmacopsychiatry 10:24–36, 1975

Gitlin MJ, Cochran SD, Jamison KR: Maintenance lithium treatment: side effects and compliance. J Clin Psychiatry 50:127–131, 1989

Glen A, Johnson L, Shepherd M: Continuation therapy with lithium and amitriptyline in unipolar depressive illness: a randomized double-blind, controlled trial. Psychol Med 14:37–50, 1984

Glesinger B: Evaluation of lithium in treatment of psychotic excitement. Med J Aust 41:277–283, 1954

Glue PW, Nutt DJ, Cowen PJ, et al: Selective effect of lithium on cognitive performance in man. Psychopharmacology (Berl) 91:109–111, 1987

Godfrey PP: Potentiation by lithium of CMP-phosphatidate formation in carbachol-stimulated rat cerebral-cortical slices and its reversal by myoinositol. Biochem J 258:621–624, 1989

Godfrey PP, McClue SJ, White AM, et al: Subacute and chronic in vivo lithium treatment inhibits agonist- and sodium flouoride-stimulated inositol phosphate production in rat cortex. J Neurochem 52:498–506, 1989

Goldney RD, Spence ND: Safety of the combination of lithium and neuroleptic drugs. Am J Psychiatry 143:882–884, 1986

Goodnick PJ, Shapiro B: Mechanisms of lithium action: neurotransmitter balance: human studies. Rev Contemp Pharmacother 4:293–295, 1993

Goodnick PJ, Fieve RR, Schlegel A, et al: Predictors of interepisode symptoms and relapse in affective disorder patients treated with lithium carbonate. Am J Psychiatry 144:367–369, 1987

Goodwin FK, Ebert MH: Lithium in mania: clinical trials and controlled studies, in Lithium: Its Role in Psychiatric Research and Treatment. Edited by Gershon S, Shopsin B. New York, Plenum Press, 1973, pp 237–252

Goodwin FK, Jamison KR: Manic Depressive Illness. New York, Oxford University Press, 1990

Goodwin FK, Zis AP: Lithium in the treatment of mania: comparison with neuroleptics. Arch Gen Psychiatry 36:840–844, 1979

Goodwin FK, Murphy DL, Bunney WE Jr: Lithium carbonate treatment in depression and mania: a longitudinal double-blind study. Arch Gen Psychiatry 21:486–496, 1969

Goodwin FK, Murphy DL, Dunner DL, et al: Lithium response in unipolar vs. bipolar depression. Am J Psychiatry 129:44–47, 1972

Greco FA, Brereton JD: Effect of lithium carbonate on the neutropenia caused by chemotherapy: a preliminary clinical trial. Oncology 34:153–155, 1977

Greene DA, Lattimer SA: Impaired energy utilization and Na-K-ATPase in diabetic peripheral nerve. Am J Physiol 246: E311–E318, 1984

Greene DA, DeJesus PV, Winegard AI: Effects of insulin and dietary myo-inositol on impaired peripheral motor nerve conduction velocity in acute streptozotocin diabetes. J Clin Invest 55:1326–1336, 1975

Greene DA, Lattimer SA, Sima AAF: Sorbitol, phosphoinositides, and sodium-potassium-ATPase in the pathogenesis of diabetic complications. N Engl J Med 316:599–606, 1987

Greenhill LL, Rieder RO, Wender PH, et al: Lithium carbonate in the treatment of hyperactive children. Arch Gen Psychiatry 28:636–640, 1973

Greenspan K, Goodwin FK, Bunney WE, et al: Lithium ion retention and distribution. Arch Gen Psychiatry 19:664–673, 1968a

Greenspan K, Green R, Durell J: Retention and distribution patterns of lithium, a pharmacological tool in studying the pathophysiology of manic-depressive psychosis. Am J Psychiatry 125:512, 519, 1968b

Greenspan K, Aronoff MS, Bogdanski DF: Effects of lithium carbonate on turnover and metabolism of norepinephrine in rat brain-correlation to gross behavioral effects. Pharmacol Biochem Behav 3:129–136, 1970a

Greenspan K, Schildkraut JJ, Gordon EK, et al: Catecholamine metabolism in affective disorders, III: MHPG and other catecholamine metabolites in patients treated with lithium carbonate. J Psychiatr Res 7:171–183, 1970b

Groth U, Prellwitz W, Jahnchen E: Estimation of pharmacokinetic parameters of lithium from saliva and urine. Clin Pharmacol Ther 16:490–498, 1974

Growe GA, Crayton JW, Klass DB, et al: Lithium in chronic schizophrenia. Am J Psychiatry 136:454–455, 1979

Gupta JD, Crollini C: Effect of lithium on magnesium-dependent enzymes. Lancet 2:225–226, 1974

Gupta RC, Robinson WA, Kurnick JE: Felty's syndrome: effect of lithium on granulopoiesis. Am J Med 61:29–32, 1976

Gusovsky F, Hollingsworth EB, Daly JW: Regulation of phosphatidylinositol turnover in brain synaptoneurosomes: stimulatory effects of agents that enhance influx of sodium ions. Proc Natl Acad Sci USA 83:3003–3007, 1986

Gusovsky F, Hollingsworth EB, Daly JW: Stimulation of phosphoinositide breakdown in brain synaptoneurosomes by agents that activate sodium influx: antagonism by tetrodotoxin, saxitoxin and cadmium. Mol Pharmacol 32:479–487, 1987

Gyulai L, Bolinger L, Leigh JS Jr, et al: Phosphorylethanolamine—the major constituent of the phosphomonoester peak observed by ^{31}P-NMR on developing dog brain. FEBS Lett 178:137–142, 1984

Haas M, Schooler J, Tosteson DC: Coupling of lithium to sodium transport in human red cells. Nature 258:425–427, 1975

Hale MS, Donaldson JO: Lithium carbonate in the treatment of organic brain syndrome. J Nerv Ment Dis 170:362–365, 1982

Hallcher LM, Sherman WR: The effects of lithium ion and other agents on the activity of myoinositol-1-phosphatase from bovine brain. J Biol Chem 255:10896–10901, 1980

Hamlyn JM, Blaustein MP, Bova S, et al: Identification and characterization of a ouabain-like compound from human plasma. Proc Natl Acad Sci USA 88:6259–6263, 1991

Hansen CA, Siemens IR, Williamson JR: Calcium entry in rat hepatocytes: stimulation by inositol 1,4,5-trisphosphothioate, in The Biology and Medicine of Signal Transduction. Edited by Nishizuka Y, et al. New York, Raven Press, 1990, pp 128–133

Hansen HE, Amdisen A: Lithium intoxication. Quarterly Journal of Medicine (New Series) 47:123–144, 1978

Hansen HE, Hestbech J, Sorensen JL, et al: Chronic interstitial nephropathy in patients on long-term lithium treatment. Quarterly Journal of Medicine New Series 48:577–591, 1979

Harrison CD, Cooper G, Zujko KF, et al: Myocardial and mitochondrial function in potassium depletion cardiomyopathy. J Mol Cell Cardiol 4:633–649, 1972

Hartigan GP: The use of lithium salts in affective disorders. Br J Psychiatry 109:810–814, 1963

Hartley CE: The effect of lithium on Herpes Simplex virus replication. Med Lab Sci 40:406–408, 1983

Harvey B, Carstens M, Taljaard J: Mechanisms of lithium action: essential fatty acids. Rev Contemp Pharmacother 4:312–314, 1993

Haskovec L, Rysanek K: Die Wirkung von Lithium auf den metabolismus der Katecholamine und Indolalkylamine beim Menschen. Arzeneimittel-Forsch 19:426–427, 1969

Hasstedt SJ, Wu LL, Ash KO, et al: Hypertension and sodium-lithium countertransport in Utah pedigrees: evidence for major-locus inheritance. Am J Hum Genet 43:14–22, 1988

Hauser G: Myoinositol transport in slices of rat kidney cortex, I: effect of incubation conditions and inhibitors. Biochim Biophys Acta 173:257–266, 1969

Hedley JM, Turner JG, Brownie BEW, et al: Low dose lithium-cabimazole in the treatment of thyrotoxicosis. Aust NZJ Med 8:628–630, 1978

Heninger GR, Charney DS, Sternberg DE: Lithium carbonate augmentation of antidepressant treatment: an effective prescription for treatment-refractory depression. Arch Gen Psychiatry 40:1335–1342, 1983

Hesketh JE: Changes in membrane adenosine triphosphatases on administration of lithium salts in vivo. Biochem Soc Trans 4:328–330, 1976

Hesketh JE, Glen AIM, Reading HW: Membrane ATPase activities in depressive illness. J Neurochem 28:1401–1402, 1977

Hesketh JE, Loudon JB, Reading HW, et al: The effect of lithium treatment on erythrocyte membrane ATPase activities and erythrocyte ion content. Br J Clin Pharmacol 5:323–329, 1978

Hestbech J, Aurell M: Lithium-induced uremia. Lancet 1:212–213, 1979

Hestbech J, Hansen HE, Amdisen A, et al: Chronic renal lesions following long-term treatment with lithium. Kidney Int 12:205–213, 1977

Heaurteaux C, Baumann N, Lachapelle F, et al: Lithium distribution in the brain of normal mice and of "quaking" dysmyelinating mutants. J Neurochem 46:1317–1321, 1986

Hewick DS, Murray N: Red-blood-cell levels and lithium toxicity (letter). Lancet 2:473, 1976

Hiatt A, McDonough AA, Edelman IS: Assembly of the (NA^+,K^+)-adenosine triphosphatase. Post-translational membrane integration of the α-subunit. J Biol Chem 259:2629–2635, 1984

Hibbeln JR, Palmer JW, Davis JM: Are disturbances in lipid-protein interactions by phospholipase A_2 a predisposing factor in affective illness? Biol Psychiatry 25:945–961, 1989

Higashijima T, Ferguson, KM, Sternweis PC, et al: Effects of Mg^{2+} and the βδ-subunit complex on the interactions of guanine nucleotides with G proteins. J Biol Chem 262:762–766, 1987

Hill G, Jacobs KH: Activation of cardiac G proteins by muscarinic acetylcholine receptors: regulation by Mg^{2+} and Na^+ ions. Eur J Pharmacol 172:155–163, 1989

Hill TD, Dean NM, Boynton AL: Inositol 1,3,4,5-tetrakisphosphate induces Ca^{2+} sequestration in rat liver cells. Science 242:1176–1178, 1988

Himmelhoch JM, Garfinkel ME: Sources of lithium resistance in mixed mania. Psychopharmacol Bull 22:613–620, 1986

Himmelhoch JM, Detre T, Kupfer DJ, et al: Treatment of previously intractable depressions with tranylcypromine and lithium. J Nerv Ment Dis 155:216–220, 1972

Himmelhoch JM, Poust RI, Mallinger AG, et al: Adjustment of lithium dose during lithium-chlorothiazide therapy. Clin Pharmacol Ther 22:225–227, 1977a

Himmelhoch JM, Rorrest J, Neil JF, et al: Thiazide-lithium synergy in refractory mood swings. Am J Psychiatry 134:149–152, 1977b

Hirata Y, Okada K: Relation of NA^+,K^+-ATPase to delayed motor nerve conduction velocity: effect of aldose reductase inhibitor, ADN-138, on NA^+,K^+-ATPase activity. Metabolism 39:563–567, 1990

Hirschowitz J, Casper R, Garver DL, et al: Lithium response in good prognosis schizophrenia. Am J Psychiatry 137:916–920, 1980

Hirvonen M-R: Cerebral lithium, inositol and inositol monophosphates. Pharmacol Toxicol 69:22–27, 1991

Ho AKS, Loh HH, Craves F, et al: The effect of prolonged lithium treatment on the synthesis rate and turnover of monoamines in brain regions of rats. Eur J Pharmacol 10:72–78, 1970

Hodgkin AL: The Conduction of the Nervous Impulse. Springfield, IL, Charles C. Thomas, 1964

Hokin-Neaverson M, Jefferson JW: Deficient erythrocyte Na,K-ATPase activity in different affective states in bipolar affective disorder and normalization by lithium therapy. Neuropsychobiology 22:18–25, 1989a

Hokin-Neaverson M, Jefferson JW: Erythrocyte sodium pump activity in bipolar affective disorder and other psychiatric disorders. Neuropsychobiology 11:1–7, 1989b

Hokin-Neaverson M, Spiegel DA, Lewis WC: Deficiency of erythrocyte sodium pump activity in bipolar manic-depressive psychosis. Life Sci 15:1739–1748, 1974

Hokin-Neaverson M, Spiegel DA, Lewis WC, et al: Erythrocyte sodium pump activity in different psychiatric disorders. Research Communications in Psychology Psychiatry & Behavior 3:391–403, 1976

Honchar MP, Olney JW, Sherman WR: Systemic cholinergic agents induce seizures and brain damage in lithium-treated rats. Science 220:323–325, 1983

Honchar MP, Ackermann KE, Sherman WR: Chronically administered lithium alters neither myoinositol monophosphatase activity nor phosphoinositide levels in rat brain. J Neurochem 53:590–594, 1989

Honchar MP, Vogler GP, Gish BG, et al: Evidence that phosphoinositide metabolism in rat cerebral cortex stimulated by pilocarpine, physostigmine, and pargyline in vivo is not changed by chronic lithium treatment. J Neurochem 55:1521–1525, 1990

Hope PL, Costello AM, Cady EB, et al: Cerebral energy metabolism studied with phosphorus NMR spectroscopy in normal and birth asphyxiated infants. Lancet 2:366–370, 1984

Horisberger J-D, Lemas V, Kraehenbuhl J-P, et al: Structure-function relationship of Na,K-ATPase. Annu Rev Physiol 53:565–584, 1991

Horrobin DF: Lithium, fatty acids and seborrhoeic dermatitis: a new mechanism of lithium action and a new treatment for seborrhoeic dermatitis. Lithium 1:149–155, 1990

House C, Kemp BE: Protein kinase C contains a pseudosubstrate prototype in its regulatory domain. Science 238:1726–1728, 1987

Hullin RP, McDonald R, Allsopp MNE: Prophylactic lithium in recurrent affective disorders. Lancet 1:1044–1046, 1972

Hullin RP, McDonald R, Allsopp MNE: Further report on prophylactic lithium in recurrent affective disorders. Br J Psychiatry 126:281–284, 1975

Hullin RP, Coley VP, Birch NJ, et al: Renal function after long-term treatment with lithium. Br Med J 1:1457–1459, 1979

Issac G: Bipolar disorder in prepubertal children. J Clin Psychiatry 52(4):165–168, 1991

Issac G: Misdiagnosed bipolar disorder in adolescents in a special educational school and treatment program. J Clin Psychiatry 53:133–136, 1992

Itil TM, Akpinar S: Lithium effect on human electroencephalogram. Clin Electroencephalogr 2:89–102, 1971

Iyengar R, Birnbaumer L: Hormone receptor modulates the regulatory component of adenylyl cyclase by reducing its requirement for Mg^{2+} and enhancing its extent of activation by quanine nucleotides. Proc Natl Acad Sci USA 79:5179–5183, 1982

Jacob Al, Hope RR: Prolongation of Q-T interval in lithium toxicity. Electrocardiology 12:117–119, 1979

Jaffe CM: First degree atrioventricular block during lithium carbonate treatment. Am J Psychiatry 134:88–89, 1977

Janis RA, Silver PJ, Triggle DJ: Drug action and cellular calcium regulation. Adv Drug Res 16:309–591, 1987

Janowsky DS, El-Yousef MK, Davis JM, et al: A cholinergic-adrenergic hypothesis of mania and depression. Lancet 2:632–635, 1972

Janowsky DS, El-Yousef MK, Davis JM, et al: Parasympathetic suppression of manic symptoms by physostigmine. Arch Gen Psychiatry 28:542–547, 1973

Jefferson JW: Lithium: a therapeutic magic wand. J Clin Psychiatry 50:81–86, 1989

Jenkins RJ, Aronson JK, Brearley CJ: Increases in Na/K pump numbers in isolated human lymphocytes exposed to lithium in vitro: reversal by myoinositol and by inhibitors of protein kinase C and the Na/H antiport. Biochim Biophys Acta 1092:138–144, 1991

Jenner FA, Lee CR: Intracellular lithium and clinical response. Lancet 2:641–642, 1976

Joffe RT, Kellner CH, Post RM, et al: Lithium increases platelet count (letter). N Engl J Med 311:674, 1984

Joffe RT, Singer W, Levitt AJ, et al: A placebo-controlled comparison of lithium and triiodothyronine augmentation of tricyclic antidepressants in unipolar refractory depression. Arch Gen Psychiatry 50:387–393, 1993

Johnson FN: The History of Lithium Therapy. London, MacMillan, 1984

Johnson G: Lithium and EEG: an analysis of behavioral, biochemical, and electrographic changes. Electroencephalogr Clin Neurophysiol 29:656–657, 1969

Johnson G: Antidepressant effect of lithium. Compr Psychiat 15:43–47, 1974

Johnson G, Gershon S, Hekimian LJ: Controlled evaluation of lithium and chlorpromazine in the treatment of manic states: an interim report. Compr Psychiatry 9:563–573, 1968

Johnson G, Maecario M, Gershon S, et al: The effects of lithium on electroencephalogram, behavior and serum electrolytes. J Nerv Ment Dis 151:273–289, 1970

Johnson GF: Lithium neurotoxicity. Aust N Z J Psychiatry 10:33–38, 1976

Johnston BB, Naylor GJ, Dick EG, et al: Prediction of clinical course of bipolar manic depressive illness treated with lithium. Psychol Med 10:329–334, 1980

Jones F-Del, Maas JW, Dekirmenjian H, et al: Urinary catecholamine metabolites during behavioral changes in a patient with manic depressive cycles. Science 179:300–302, 1973

Jorkasky D, Amsterdam J, Cox M: Lithium induced nephropathy: a 3 year prospective study. Kidney Int 27:141–144, 1985

Joseph NE, Renshaw PF, Leight JS Jr: Systemic lithium administration alters rat cerebral cortex phospholipids. Biol Psychiatry 22:540–544, 1987

Joseph SK, Rice HL: The relationship between inositol triphosphate receptor density and calcium release in brain microsomes. Mol Pharmacol 35:355–359, 1989

Kallen B, Tandberg A: Lithium and pregnancy: a cohort study on manic-depressive women. Acta Psychiatr Scand 68:134–139, 1983

Kane JM: The role of neuroleptics in manic-depressive illness. J Clin Psychiatry 49(suppl 1):12–13, 1988

Kantor D, McNevin S, Leichner P, et al: The benefit of lithium carbonate adjunct in refractory depression: fact or fiction? Can J Psychiatry 31:583–588, 1982

Kato T, Shioiri T, Takahashi S, et al: Measurement of brain phosphoinositide metabolism in bipolar patients using in vivo [31] P-MRS. J Affect Disord 22:185–190, 1991

Katz B, Miledi R: Ionic requirements of synaptic transmitter release. Nature 215:651–655, 1967a

Katz B, Miledi R: The release of acetylcholine from nerve endings by graded electric pulses. Proc R Soc Lond [Biol] 167:23–38, 1967b

Katz B, Miledi R: A study of synaptic transmission in the absence of nerve impulses. J Physiol (Lond) 192:407–436, 1967c

Kebabian JW, Calne DB: Multiple receptors for dopamine. Nature 277:93–96, 1979

Keller MB, Lavori PW, Coryell W, et al: Differential outcome of pure manic, mixed/cycling, and pure depressive episodes in patients with bipolar illness. JAMA 255:3138–3142, 1986

Keller MB, Lavori PW, Kane JM, et al: Subsyndromal symptoms in bipolar disorder: a comparison of standard and low serum levels of lithium. Arch Gen Psychiatry 49:371–376, 1992

Kemp BE, Pearson RB: Protein kinase recognition sequence motifs. Trends Biochem Sci 15:342–346, 1990

Kemp BE, Bylund DV, Huang TS, et al: Substrate specificity of the cAMP-dependent protein kinase. Proc Natl Acad Sci USA 72:3448–3452, 1975

Kemp BE, Pearson RB, House C, et al: Regulation of protein kinases by pseudosubstrate prototypes. Cell Signal 1:303–311, 1989

Kendall DA, Nahorski SR: Acute and chronic lithium treatments influence agonist and depolarization-stimulated inositol phospholipid hydrolysis in rat cerebral cortex. J Pharmacol Exp Therap 241:1023–1027, 1987

Kennedy ED, Challiss RA, Ragan CI, et al: Reduced inositol polyphosphate accumulation and inositol supply induced by lithium in stimulated cerebral cortex slices. Biochem J 267:781–786, 1990

Kerbeshian J, Burd L, Risher W: Lithium carbonate in the treatment of two patients with infantile autism and atypical bipolar symptomatology. J Clin Psychopharmacol 7:401–405, 1987

Kerry RJ, Liebling LI, Owen G: Weight changes in lithium responders. Acta Psychiatr Scand 46:238–243, 1979

Khan AA, Steiner JP, Klein MG, et al: IP_3 receptor: localization to plasma membrane of T cells and cocapping with the T cell receptor. Science 257:815–818, 1992

Khan MC: Lithium carbonate in the treatment of acute depressive illness. Bibl Psychiatr 161:244–248, 1981

Kim J, Jyrizai H, Greene DA: Normalization of NA⁺-K⁺-ATPase activity in isolated membrane fraction from sciatic nerves of streptozotocin-induced diabetic rats by dietary myoinositol supplementation in vivo or protein kinase C agonists in vitro. Diabetes 40:558–567, 1991a

Kim J, Rushovich EH, Thomas TP, et al: Diminished specific activity of cytosolic protein kinase C in sciatic nerve of streptozocin-induced diabetic rats and its correction by dietary myoinositol. Diabetes 40:1545–1554, 1991b

Kincaid-Smith P, Burrows GD, Davies DM, et al: Renal biopsy findings in lithium and pre-lithium patients. Lancet 2:700–701, 1979

Kingstone E: The lithium treatment of hypomanic and manic states. Compr Psychiatry 11:317–320, 1960

Klein E, Patel J, Zohar J: Chronic lithium treatment increases the phosphorylation of a 64k protein in rat brain. Brain Res 407:312–316, 1987

Klein R, Praque MD, Nunn RF: Clinical and biochemical analysis of a case of manic-depressive psychosis showing regular weekly cycles. Journal of Mental Science 91:79–88, 1945

Kline NS: Lithium: the history of its use in psychiatry. Mod Probl Pharmacopsychiatry 3:75–92, 1969

Kline NS, Wren JC, Cooper TB, et al: Evaluation of lithium therapy in chronic and periodic alcoholism. Am J Med Sci 168:15–22, 1974

Knapp S, Mandell AJ: Short- and long-term lithium administration: effects on brain's serotonergic biosynthetic systems. Science 180:645–647, 1973

Knorring L, Oreland L, Perris C, et al: Evaluation of the lithium RBC/plasma ratio as a predictor of the prophylactic effect of lithium treatment in affective disorders. Pharmakopsychiatrie 9:81–84, 1976

Knudsen GM, Jakobsen J, Barry DI, et al: Myoinositol normalizes decreased sodium permeability of the blood-brain barrier in streptozotocin diabetes. Neuroscience 29:773–777, 1989

Kofman O, Belmaker RH: Intracerebroventricular myoinositol antagonizes lithium-induced suppression of rearing behavior in rats. Brain Res 534:345–347, 1990

Kohn PG, Clausen T: The relationship between the transport of glucose and cations across cell membranes in isolated tissues. Biochim Biophys Acta 255:798–814, 1972

Kranzler HR, Liebowitz NR: Anxiety and depression in substance abuse: clinical implications. Med Clin North Am 72:867–885, 1988

Kudrow L: Lithium prophylaxis for chronic cluster headache. Headache 17:15–18, 1977

Kudrow W: Cluster Headache: Mechanisms and Management. New York, Oxford University Press, 1980

Kuffler SW, Nicholl JC: From Neuron to Brain, 2nd Edition. New York Oxford University Press, 1979

Kutcher SP, Marton P, Korenblum M: Relationship between psychiatric illness and conduct disorder in adolescents. Can J Psychiatry 42:937–947, 1989

Labelle A, Lapierre YD: Keratodermia: side effects of lithium. J Clin Psychopharmacol 11:149–150, 1991

Lai Y, Nairn AC, Greengard P: Autophosphorylation reversibly regulates the Ca^{2+}/calmodulin-dependence of Ca^{2+}/calmodulin/dependent protein kinase II. Proc Natl Acad Sci USA 83:4253–4257, 1986

Lassen UV: Membrane potential and membrane resistance of red cells, in Oxygen Affinity of Hemoglobin and Red Cell Acid Base States. Edited by Roth M, Astrup P. New York, Academic Press, 1972, pp 291–304

Lavender S, Brown JN, Berrill WT: Acute renal failure and lithium intoxication. Postgrad Med J 49:277–279, 1973

Lazarus JH, McGregor AM, Ludgate M, et al: Effect of lithium carbonate therapy on thyroid immune status in manic depressive patients: a prospective study. J Affect Disord 11:155–160, 1986

Lazarus LH, Kitron N: Depression of D.N.A.-polymerase activity by lithium. Lancet 2:225–226, 1974

Lederer WJ, Nelson MT: Sodium pump stoichiometry determined by simultaneous measurements of sodium efflux and membrane current in barnacle. J Physiol (Lond) 348:665–667, 1984

Lee TS, MacGregor LC, Fluharty SJ, et al: Differential regulation of protein kinase C and (Na,K)-adenosine triphosphatase activities by elevated glucose levels in retinal capillary endothelial cells. J Clin Invest 83:90–94, 1989

Lenox RH, Watson DG: Lithium and the brain: a psychopharmacological strategy to a molecular basis for manic depressive illness. Clin Chem 40:309–314, 1994

Lenox RH, Newhouse PA, Creelman WL, et al: Adjunctive treatment of manic agitation with lorazepam versus haloperidol: a double-blind study. J Clin Psychiatry 53:47–52, 1992

Leonard DP, Kidson MA, Shannon PJ, et al: Double-blind trial of lithium carbonate and haloperidol in Huntington's chorea. Lancet 2:1208–1209, 1974

Lerer B, Stanley M: Effect of chronic lithium on cholinergically mediated responses and [^{3}H]QNB binding in rat brain. Brain Res 344:211–219, 1985

Leroy M-C, Villeneuve A, LaJenunesse C: Lithium, thyroid function and antithyroid antibodies. Prog Neuropsychopharmacol Biol Psychiatry 12:483–490, 1988

Levy A, Zohar J, Belmaker RH: The effect of chronic lithium pretreatment on rat brain muscarinic receptor regulation. Neuropharmacology 21:1199–1201, 1983

Lewis DA: Lithium, internal medicine and psychiatry: an outline. J Clin Psychiatry 43:314–320, 1982

Lewis DA, Bacher NM, Field PB: Addition of lithium to neuroleptic treatment in chronic schizophrenia (letter). Am J Psychiatry 143:262, 1986

Li R, Wing LL, Wyatt RJ, et al: Effects of haloperidol, lithium, and valproate on phosphoinositide turnover in rat brain. Pharmacol Biochem Behav 46:323–329, 1993

Lieb J: Remission of recurrent herpes infection during therapy with lithium (letter). N Engl J Med 301:942, 1979

Lieberman KW, Stoeks PE, van der Noot G: Lithium metabolism and intracellular electrolytes. Brain Res Bull 3:414–418, 1978

Lindstedt G, Nilsson L, Walinder J, et al: On the prevalence, diagnosis, and management of lithium-induced hypothyroidism in psychiatric patients. Br J Psychiatry 130:452–458, 1977

Lingjaerde O, Edlund AH, Gormsen CA, et al: The effect of lithium carbonate in combination with tricyclic antidepressants in endogenous depression: a double-blind, multicenter trial. Acta Psychiatr Scand 50:233–242, 1974

Linnoila M, MacDonald E, Reinila M, et al: RBC membrane adenosine triphosphatase activities in patients with major affective disorders. Arch Gen Psychiatry 40:1021–1026, 1983

Lippmann S: Is lithium bad for the kidney? J Clin Psychiatry 43:220–224, 1982

Lippmann S, Wagemaker H, Tucker D: A practical approach to management of lithium concurrent with hyponatremia, diuretic therapy and/ or chronic failure. J Clin Psychiatry 42:304–306, 1981

Lou LL, Lloyd SJ, Schulman H: Activation of the multifunctional Ca^{2+}/ calmodulin-dependent protein kinase by autophosphorylation: ATP modulates production of an autonomous enzyme. Proc Natl Acad Sci USA 83:9497–9501, 1986

Louie AK, Meltzer HY: Lithium potentation of antidepressant treatment. J Clin Psychopharmacol 4:316–321, 1984

Lu KM, Zhong XL, Zhu XX, et al: [Alterations in the sorbitol pathway and the NA^+- K^+-ATPase activity of peripheral nerve of alloxan-induced diabetic rats]. (Chinese). Sheng Li Hsueh Pao—Acta Physiologia Sinica 42:401–405, 1990

Luchins DJ, Kojka D: Lithium and propranolol in aggression and self-injurious behavior in the mentally retarded. Psychopharmacol Bull 25:372–375, 1989

Lyman GH, Williams CC, Preston D: The use of lithium carbonate to reduce infection and leukopenia during systemic chemotherapy. N Engl J Med 302:257–260, 1980

Lyskowski J, Narallah HA, Dunner FJ, et al: A longitudinal survey of side effects in a lithium clinic. J Clin Psychiatry 43:284–286, 1982

Maas JW: Biogenic amines and depression: biochemical and pharmacologic separation of two types of depression. Arch Gen Psychiatry 32:1357–1361, 1975

Mackay AVP, Sheppard GP, Saha BK, et al: Failure of lithium treatment in established tardive dyskinesia. Psychol Med 10:583–587, 1980

Madakasira S: Low dose potency of lithium in antidepressant augmentation. Psychiatr J Univ Ott 11:107–109, 1986

Maeda N, Kawasaki T, Nakade S, et al: Structural and functional characterization of inositol 1,4,5-triphosphate receptor channel from mouse cerebellum. J Biol Chem 266:1109–1116, 1991

Maggi A, Enna SJ: Regional alterations in rat brain neurotransmitter systems following chronic lithium treatment. J Neurochem 34:888–892, 1982

Maggs R: Treatment of manic illness with lithium carbonate. Br J Psychiatry 109:56–65, 1963

Maj M: Effectiveness of lithium prophylaxis in schizoaffective psychoses: application of a polydiagnostic approach. Acta Psychiatr Scand 70:228–234, 1984

Maj M: Lithium prophylaxis of schizoaffective disorders: a prospective study. J Affect Disord 14:129–135, 1988

Maj M, del Vecchio M, Starage F, et al: Prediction of affective psychoses response to lithium prophylaxis. Acta Psychiatr Scand 69:37–44, 1984

Maj M, Arena F, Lovero M, et al: Factors associated with response to lithium prophylaxis in DSM III major depression and bipolar disorder. Pharmacopsychiatry 18:309–313, 1985

Maj M, Pirozzi R, Magliano L: Nonresponse to reinstituted lithium prophylaxis in previously responsive bipolar patients: prevalance and predictors. Am J Psychiatry 152:1810–1811, 1995

Mallette LE, Eichhort E: Effects of lithium carbonate on human calcium metabolism. Arch Intern Med 146:770–776, 1986

Mandersloot JG, Roelofsen B, DeGier J: Phosphatidylinositol as the endogenous activator of the $Na^+ + K^+$-ATPase in microsomes of rabbit kidney. Biochim Biophys Acta 508:478–485, 1978

Manji HK, Potter WZ, Lenox RH: Signal transduction pathways: molecular targets for lithium's actions. Arch Gen Psychiatry 52:531–543, 1995

Mannisto P, Koivisto V: Antidiabetic effects of lithium (letter). Lancet 2:1031, 1972

Mannisto PT: Endocrine side effects of lithium, in Handbook of Lithium Therapy. Edited by Johnson FN. Baltimore, MD, University Park Press, 1980, pp 289–309

Manocha M, Chokroverty S, Nora R: Peripheral and central neural conduction in patients on chronic lithium therapy. Muscle Nerve 7:575–576, 1984

Manyam NVB, Bravo-Fernandez E: Lithium carbonate in Huntington's chorea (letter). Lancet 1:1010, 1973

Margolis RU, Press R, Altszuler N, et al: Inositol production by the brain in normal and alloxan-diabetic dogs. Brain Res 28:535–539, 1971

Martin AR: Quantal nature of synaptic transmission. Physiol Rev 46:51–56, 1966

Mateer JR, Clark MR: Lithium toxicity with rarely reported ECG manifestations. Ann Emerg Med 11:208–211, 1982

Mathé AA, Theodorsson E, Stenforis C: Mechanisms of lithium action: neuropeptides. Rev Contemp Pharmacother 4 299–300, 1993

Mattsson B: Huntington's chorea and lithium therapy. Lancet 1:718–719, 1973

Mattsson B, Schoultz BV: A comparison between lithium placebo and a diuretic in premenstrual tension. Acta Psychiatr Scand Suppl 255:75–84, 1974

Mauritson DR, Winniford MD, Walker WS, et al: Oral verapamil for paroxysmal supraventricular tachycardia: a long-term, double-blind randomized trial. Ann Intern Med 96:409–412, 1982

Mayfield D, Brown RG: The clinical laboratory and electroencephalographic effects of lithium. J Psychiatr Res 4:207–219, 1966

McCarren M, Potter BVL, Miller RJ: A metabolically stable analog of 1,4,5-inositol triphosphate activates a novel K^+ conductance in pyramidal cells of the rat hippocampal slice. Neuron 3:461–471, 1989

McElroy SL, Keck PE Jr, Pope HG Jr, et al: Valproate in the treatment of rapid-cycling bipolar disorder. J Clin Psychopharmacol 8:275–279, 1988

McElroy SL, Dessain EC, Pope HG Jr, et al: Clozapine in the treatment of psychotic mood disorders, schizoaffective disorder, and schizophrenia. J Clin Psychiatry 52:411–414, 1991

McGoon MD, Vlietstra RE, Holmes RE Jr, et al: The clinical use of verapamil. Mayo Clin Proc 57:495–510, 1982

McIntosh WB, Horn EH, Mathieson LM: The prevalence, mechanism and clinical significance of lithium-induced hypercalcemia. Med Lab Sci 44:115–118, 1987

Mehta DB: Lithium and affective disorders associated with organic brain impairment (letter). Am J Psychiatry 133:236, 1976

Melia PI: Prophylactic lithium: a double-blind trial in recurrent affective disorders. Br J Psychiatry 116:621–624, 1970

Mellerup ET, Thomsen HG, Plenge P, et al: Lithium effect on plasma glucagon, liver phosphorylase-*a*, and liver glycogen in rats. J Psychiatr Res 8:37–42, 1970

Meltzer HL: Effects of lithium on intracellular calcium-mediated enzymes. Lithium 1:203–208, 1990a

Meltzer HL: Mode of action of lithium in affective disorders: an influence on intracellular calcium functions. Pharmacol Toxicol 66 (suppl 3):84–99, 1990b

Meltzer HL: Mechanism of lithium action: calcium. Reviews in Contemporary Pharmacotherapy 4:289–290, 1993

Meltzer HL, Kassir S: Abnormal calmodulin-activated Ca ATPase in manic-depressive subjects. J Psychiatr Res 17:29–35, 1983

Meltzer HL, Kassir S, Dunner DL, et al: Repression of a lithium pump as a consequence of lithium ingestion by manic-depressive subjects. Psychopharmacology 54:113–118, 1977

Meltzer HL, Kassir S, Goodnick PJ, et al: Calmodulin-activated calcium ATPase in affective disorders. Neuropsycho Biology 20:169–173, 1988

Mendels J: Relationship between depression and mania (letter). Lancet 1:342, 1971

Mendels J: Lithium in the acute treatment of depressive states, in Lithium Research and Therapy. Edited by Johnson FN. London, Academic Press, 1975, pp 43–62

Mendels J, Frazer A: Intracellular lithium concentration and clinical response: towards a membrane theory of depression. J Psychiatr Res 10:9–18, 1973

Mendels J, Frazer A, Secunda SK: Intraerythrocyte sodium and potassium in manic-depressive illness. Biol Psychiatry 5:165–171, 1972a

Mendels J, Secunda SK, Dyson WL: A controlled study of the antidepressant effects of lithium carbonate. Arch Gen Psychiatry 26:154–157, 1972b

Mendels J, Frazer A, Baron J, et al: Intra-erythrocyte lithium ion concentration and long-term maintenance treatment (letter). Lancet 1:966, 1976

Messiha FS, Agallianos D, Clower C: Dopamine excretion in affective states and following lithium$_2$ CO$_3$ therapy. Nature 225:868–869, 1970

Meyer T, Holowka D, Stryer L: Highly cooperative opening of calcium channels by inositol 1,4,5-triphosphate. Science 240:653–655, 1988

Miledi R: Transmitter release induced by injection of calcium ions into nerve terminals. Proc R Soc Land B 183:421–425, 1973

Miller SC, Kennedy MB: Regulation of brain type II Ca²⁺/calmodulin-dependent protein kinase by autophosphorylation: a Ca²⁺-triggered molecular switch. Cell 44:861–870, 1986

Mitchell J, MacKenzie TB: Cardiac effects of lithium therapy in man: a review. J Clin Psychiatry 43:47–51, 1982

Modell JG, Lenox RH, Weiner S: Inpatient clinical trial of lorazepam for the management of manic agitation. J Clin Psychopharmacol 5:109–113, 1985

Modestin J, Schwartz RB, Hunger J: [Investigation about an influence of physostigmine on schizophrenic symptoms]. Pharmakopsychiatr Neuropsychopharmakol 6:300–304, 1973

Moore RY: Catecholamine neuron systems in brain. Am Neurol 12:321–327, 1982

Mork A, Geisler A: Effects of lithium ex vivo on the GTP-mediated inhibition of calcium-stimulated adenylate cyclase activity in rat brain. Eur J Pharmacol 168:347–454, 1989

Motohashi N: Mechanisms of lithium action: GABA. Rev Contemp Pharmacother 4:299, 1993

Motohashi N, Ikawa K, Kariya T: GABA_B receptors are up-regulated by chronic treatment with lithium or carbamepine: GABA hypothesis of affective disorders? Eur J Pharmacol 166:95–99, 1989

Mukherjee S, Rosen AM, Caracci G, et al: Persistent tardive dyskinesia in bipolar patients. Arch Gen Psychiatry 43:342–346, 1986

Mumby SM, Kahn RA, Manning DR, et al: Antisera of designed specificity for subunits of guanine nucleotide-binding regulatory proteins. Proc Natl Acad Sci USA 83:265–269, 1986

Murphy DL, Brodie HK, Goodwin FK, et al: Regular induction of hypomania by L-dopa in "bipolar" manic-depressive patients. Nature 229:135–136, 1971a

Murphy DL, Goodwin FK, Bunney WE Jr: Leukocytosis during lithium treatment. Am J Psychiatry 127:1559–1561, 1971b

Myers WC, Burket RC, Otto TA: Conduct disorder and personality disorders in hospitalized adolescents. J Clin Psychiatry 54:21–26, 1993

Nahorski SR: Inositol polyphosphates and neuronal calcium homeostasis. Trends Neurosci 11:444–448, 1988

Nahorski SR, Ragan CI, Challiss RAJ: Lithium and the phosphoinositide cycle: An example of uncompetitive inhibition and its pharmacological consequences. Trend Pharmacol Sci 12:297–303, 1991

Nahunek K, Svestka J, Rodova A: Zur Stellung des Lithiums in der Gruppe der Antidepressiva in der Behandlung von akuten enogenen und Involutions depressionen [The position of lithium among antidepressants in the treatment of acute phases of endogenous and involutional depression]. Int Pharmacopsychiatry 5:249–257, 1970

Nairn AC, Hemmings HC, Greengard P: Protein kinases in the brain. Annu Rev Biochem 54:931–976, 1985

Nasr SJ, Atkins RW: Coincidental improvement in asthma during lithium treatment. Am J Psychiatry 134:1042–1043, 1977

Naylor GJ, Smith AHW: Defective genetic control of sodium-pump density in manic depressive psychosis. Psychol Med 11:257–263, 1981

Naylor GJ, McNamee HB, Moody JP: Erythrocyte sodium and potassium in depressive illness. J Psychosom Res 14:173–177, 1970

Naylor GJ, Dick DAT, Dick EG, et al: Erythrocyte membrane cation carrier in depressive illness. Psychol Med 3:502–508, 1973

Naylor GJ, Dick DAT, Dick EG, et al: Erythrocyte membrane cation carrier in mania. Psychol Med 6:659–663, 1976a

Naylor GJ, Reid AH, Dick DAT, et al: A biochemical study of short-cycle manic-depressive psychosis in mental defectives. Br J Psychiatry 128:169–180, 1976b

Naylor GJ, Smith AHW, Dick EG, et al: Erythrocyte membrane cation carrier in manic-depressive psychosis. Psychol Med 10:521–525, 1980

Naylor GJ, Corrigan FM, Smith AHW, et al: Further studies of vanadium in depressive psychosis. Br J Psychiatry 150:656–661, 1987

Neer EJ, Lok JM, Wolf LG: Purification and properties of the inhibitory guanine nucleotide regulatory unit of brain adenylate cyclase. J Biol Chem 259:14222–14229, 1984

Nelson JC, Mazure CM: Lithium augmentation in psychotic depression refractory to combined drug treatment. Am J Psychiatry 143:363–366, 1986

Newman ME, Belmaker RH: Effects of lithium in vitro and ex vivo on components of the adenylate cyclase system in membranes from the cerebral cortex of the rat. Neuropharmacology 26:211–217, 1987

Newman ME, Lichtenberg P, Belmaker RH: Effects of lithium in vitro on noradrenaline-induced cyclic AMP accumulation in rat cortical slices after reserpine-induced supersensitivity. Neuropharmacology 24:353–355, 1985

Nichols RA, Haycock JW, Wang JKT, et al: Phorbol ester enhancement of neurotransmitter release from rat brain synaptosomes. J Neurochem 48:615–621, 1987

Nielsen JL, Christensen MS, Pedersen EB: Parathyroid hormone in serum during lithium therapy. Scand J Clin Lab Invest 37:369–372, 1977

Nishizuka Y: The molecular heterogeneity of protein kinase C and its implications for cellular regulation. Nature 334:661–665, 1988

Noack CH, Trautner EM: The lithium treatment of maniacal psychosis. Med J Aust 38:219–222, 1951

Noguchi S, Mishina M, Kawamura M, et al: Expression of functional (Na^+,K^+)-ATPase from cloned cDNAs. FEBS Lett 225:27–31, 1987

Nora JJ, Nora AH, Towes WH: Lithium, Ebstein's anomaly, and other congenital heart defects. Lancet 2:594–595, 1974

Noyes R Jr, Ringdahl IC, Andreasen NJC: Effect of lithium citrate on adrenocortical activity in manic-depressive illness. Compr Psychiatry 12:337–347, 1971

Noyes R Jr, Dempsey GM, Blum A: Lithium treatment of depression. Compr Psychiatry 15:187–190, 1974

Nurnberger JI: Single case study: diuretic-induced lithium toxicity presenting as mania. J Nerv Ment Dis 173:316–318, 1985

Nurnberger JI Jr, Jimerson DC, Allen JR, et al: Red cell ouabain-sensitive Na^+-K^+-adenosine triphosphatase: a state marker in affective disorder inversely related to plasma cortisol. Biol Psychiatry 17:981–992, 1982

O'Brien PM: The premenstrual syndrome: a review of the present status of therapy. Drugs 24:140–151, 1982

Olianas MC, Onali P, Neff NH, et al: Adenylate cyclase activity of synaptic membranes from rat striatum: inhibition by muscarinic receptor agonists. Mol Pharmacol 23:393–398, 1983

Oppenheim G, Ebstein RP, Belmaker RH: Effect of lithium on the physostigmine-induced behavioral syndrome and plasma cyclic GMP. J Psychiatr Res 15:133–138, 1979

Osterrieder W, Brum G, Hescheler J, et al: Injection of subunits of cyclic AMP-dependent protein kinase into cardiac myocytes modulates Ca^{2+} current. Nature 298:576–578, 1982

Ostrow DG, Pandey GN, David JM, et al: A heritable disorder of lithium transport in erythrocytes of a subpopulation of manic-depressive patients. Am J Psychiatry 135:1070–1078, 1978

Pamphlet RS, Mackenzie RA: Severe peripheral neuropathy due to lithium intoxication. J Neurol Neurosurg Psychiatry 45:656, 1982

Pandey GN, Sarkadi B, Haas M, et al: Lithium transport pathways in human red blood cells. J Gen Physiol 72:233–247, 1978

Pandey GN, Goel I, Davis JM: Effect of neuroleptic drugs on lithium uptake by the human erythrocyte. Clin Pharmacol Ther 26:96–102, 1979

Paolisso G, Sgambato S, Guidliano D, et al: Impaired insulin-induced erythrocyte magnesium accumulation is correlated to impaired insulin-mediated glucose disposal in type 2 (non-insulin-dependent) diabetic patients. Diabetologia 31:910–915, 1988

Parks DG, Greenway FL, Pack AT: Prevention of recurrent Herpes type II infection with lithium carbonate (abstract). Clin Res 36:147A, 1988

Paul MI, Ditzion BR, Janowsky DS: Affective illness and cyclic-AMP excretion (letter). Lancet 1:88, 1970a

Paul MI, Ditzion BR, Pauk GL, et al: Urinary adenosine 3′,5′-monophosphate excretion in affective disorders. Am J Psychiatry 126(10): 1493–1497, 1970b

Peatfield RC, Rose FC: Exacerbation of migraine by treatment with lithium. Headache 21:140–142, 1981

Pennefeather P, Lancaster B, Adams PR, et al: Two distinct Ca-dependent K currents in bullfrog sympathetic ganglion cells. Proc Natl Acad Sci USA 82:3040–3044, 1985

Perris C: The concept of cycloid psychotic disorder. Psychiatr Dev 1:37–56, 1988

Perry F, Sherman AD: Plasma GABA levels in psychiatric illness. J Affect Disord 6:131–138, 1984

Perry PJ, Alexander B, Prince RA, et al: The utility of a single-point dosing protocol for predicting steady-state lithium levels. Br J Psychiatry 148:401–405, 1986

Pert A, Roseblatt JE, Sivit C, et al: Long-term treatment with lithium prevents the development of dopamine receptor supersensitivity. Science 201:171–173, 1978

Peters HA: Lithium intoxication producing choreoathetosis with recovery. Wis Med J 48:1075–1076, 1949

Pi EH, Sramek JJ, Simpson GM: Effect of lithium on leukocytes: a two-year follow-up. J Clin Psychiatry 44:139–140, 1983

Piton M, Barthe M-I, Laloum D, et al: Severe lithium intoxication (presentation of two cases: a mother and her newborn son). Therapie 28:1123–1133, 1973

Platman SR, Fieve RR: The effect of lithium carbonate on the electro-encephalogram of patients with affective disorders. Br J Psychiatry 115:1185–1188, 1969

Platt JE, Campbell M, Green WH, et al: Cognitive effects of lithium carbonate and haloperidol in treatment-resistant aggressive children. Arch Gen Psychiatry 41:657–662, 1984

Plenge P, Mellerup ET, Rafaelsen OJ: Lithium action on glucogen synthesis in rat brain, liver, and diaphragm. J Psychiatr Res 8:29–36, 1970

Pope HG Jr, Lipinski JF, Cohen BM, et al: "Schizoaffective disorder": an invalid diagnosis? a comparison of schizoaffective disorder, schizophrenia, and affective disorder. Am J Psychiatry 137:921–927, 1980

Pope HG Jr, McElroy SL, Nixon RA: Possible synergism between fluoxetine and lithium in refractory depression. Am J Psychiatry 145:1292–1294, 1988

Post RM: Prophylaxis of bipolar affective disorders. International Review of Psychiatry 2:277–320, 1990

Post RM, Leverich GS, Altshuler L, et al: Lithium-discontinuation-induced refractoriness: preliminary observations. Am J Psychiatry 149:1727–1729, 1992

Potter WZ: Mechanisms of lithium action: catecholaminergic receptors. Rev Contemp Pharmacother 4:300–301, 1993

Poust RI, Mallinger AG, Mallinger J, et al: Effect of chlorothiazide on pharmacokinetics of lithium in plasma and erythrocytes. Psychopharmacol Commun 2:273–284, 1976

Prange AJ Jr: The pharmacology and biochemistry of depression. Dis Nerv Syst 25:217–221, 1964

Price LH, Conwell Y, Nelson JC: Lithium augmentation of combined neuroleptic-tricyclic treatment of delusional depression. Am J Psychiatry 140:318–322, 1983

Price LH, Charney DS, Henninger GR: Efficacy of lithium-tranylcypromine treatment in refractory depression. Am J Psychiatry 142:619–623, 1985

Price LH, Charney DS, Henninger GR: Variability of response to lithium augmentation in refractory depression. Am J Psychiatry 143:1387–1392, 1986

Price LH, Charney DS, Delgado PL, et al: Lithium and serotonin hypothesis of depression. Psychopharmacology 100:3–12, 1990

Prien RF, Caffey EM Jr, Klett CJ: Comparison of lithium carbonate and chlorpromazine in the treatment of mania. Arch Gen Psychiatry 26:146–153, 1972

Prien RF, Klett CJ, Caffey EM Jr: Lithium carbonate and imipramine in prevention of affective episodes: a comparison of recurrent affective illness. Arch Gen Psychiatry 29:420–425, 1973

Prien R, Kupfer D, Mansky P, et al: Drug therapy in prevention of recurrences in unipolar and bipolar affective disorders. Arch Gen Psychiatry 41:1096–1104, 1984

Prien RF, Himmelhoch JM, Kupfer DJ: Treatment of mixed mania. J Affect Disord 15:9–15, 1988

Pringuey D, Yzombard G, Charbit J-J, et al: Lithium kinetics during hemodialysis in a patient with lithium poisoning. Am J Psychiatry 138:249–251, 1981

Procci WR: Schizo-affective psychosis: fact or fiction? a survey of the literature. Arch Gen Psychiatry 33:1167–1178, 1976

Quitkin F, Rifkin A, Kane J, et al: Prophylactic effect of lithium and imipramine in unipolar and bipolar II patients: a preliminary report. Am J Psychiatry 135:570–572, 1978

Rabin PL, Evans DC: Exophthalmos and elevated thyroxine levels in association with lithium therapy. J Clin Psychiatry 42:398–400, 1981

Rabin EZ, Garston RG, Weir RV, et al: Persistent nephrogenic diabetes insipidus associated with long-term lithium carbonate therapy. Can Med Assoc J 121:194–198, 1979

Racker E: Fluxes of Ca²⁺ and concepts. Fed Proc 39:2422–2424, 1980

Ragan CI: The effect of lithium on inositol phosphate metabolism, in Lithium and Cell Physiology. Edited by Bach RO, Gallicchio VS. New York, Springer-Verlag, 1990, pp 102–120

Ragan CI, Watling KJ, Gee NS, et al: The dephosphorylation of inositol 1,4-biphosphate to inositol in liver and brain involves two distinct lithium⁺-sensitive enzymes and proceeds via inositol 4-phosphate. Biochem J 249:143–148, 1988

Rakowski RF, Gadsby DC, DeWeer P: Stoichiometry and voltage dependence of the sodium pump in voltage-clamped, internally dialyzed squid giant axons. J Gen Physiol 93:903–941, 1989

Ramsey TA, Frazer A, Mendels J: Plasma and erythrocyte cations in affective illness. Neuropsychobiology 5:1–10, 1979a

Ramsey TA, Frazer A, Mendels J, et al: The erythrocyte lithium-plasma lithium ratio in patients with primary affective disorder. Arch Gen Psychiatry 36:457–461, 1979b

Reda FA, Scanlan JM, Escobar JI: Treatment of tardive dyskinesia with lithium carbonate (letter). N Engl J Med 291:850, 1974

Reda FA, Escobar JI, Scanlan JM: Lithium carbonate in the treatment of tardive dyskinesia. Am J Psychiatryr 132:560–563, 1975

Reddy PL, Khanna S, Subhash MN, et al: Erythrocyte membrane Na-K-ATPase activity in affective disorder. Biol Psychiatry 26:533–537, 1989

Reddy PL, Khanna S, Subhash MN, et al: Erythrocyte membrane sodium-potassium adenosine triphosphatase activity in affective disorders. J Neural Transm Gen Sect 89:209–218, 1992

Redmann B, Jefferson JW: Lithium and Wisconsin—a medicinal trip through history. Wis Med J 84:23–26, 1985

Reed SM, Wise MG, Timmerman I: Choreoathetosis: a sign of lithium toxicity. J Neuropsychiatry 1:57–60, 1989

Rees L, Davis B: A study of the value of haloperidol in the management and treatment of schizophrenic and manic patients. Int J Neuropsychiatry 1:263–266 , 1965

Reifman A, Wyatt RJ: Lithium: a brake in the rising cost of mental illness. Arch Gen Psychiatry 37:385–388, 1980

Reisberg B, Gershon S: Side effects associated with lithium therapy. Arch Gen Psychiatry 36:879–887, 1979

Reiser G, Schäfer R, Donïe F, et al: A high-affinity inositol 1,3,4,5-tetrakisphosphate receptor protein from brain is specifically labelled by a newly synthesized photoaffinity analogue, N-(4-azidosalicyl) aminoethanol (1)-1-phospho-D-myoinositol 3,4,5-triphosphate. Biochem J 280 (Pt 2):533–539, 1991

Reiss AL: Developmental manifestations in a boy with prepubertal bipolar disorder. J Clin Psychiatry 46:441–443, 1985

Renshaw PF, Joseph NE, Leight JS Jr: Chronic dietary lithium induces increased levels of myoinositol-l-phosphatase activity in rat cerebral cortex homogenates. Brain Res 380:401–404, 1986

Rice D: The use of lithium salts in the treatment of manic states. Journal Mental Science 102:604–611, 1956

Richardson RT, DeLong MR: A reappraisal of the functions of the nucleus basalis of Meynert. Trends Neurosci 11:264–267, 1988

Richman AV, Masco HL, Rifkin SI, et al: Minimal change disease and the nephrotic syndrome associated with lithium therapy. Ann Intern Med 92:70–72, 1980

Richman CM, Makii MM, Wieser PA, et al: Effect of lithium carbonate on chemotherapy-induced neutropenia and thrombocytopenia. Am J Hematol 16:313–323, 1984

Rickels K, Feighner JP, Smith WT: A double-blind comparison of alprazolam, amitriptyline, doxepin and placebo in the treatment of major depression. Arch Gen Psychiatry 43:134–141, 1985

Rifkin A, Quitkin F, Carillo C: Lithium carbonate in emotionally unstable character disorder. Arch Gen Psychiatry 27:519–523, 1972

Roberts DE, Berman SM, Nakasatao S, et al: Effect of lithium carbonate on zidovudine-associated neutropenia in the acquired immunodeficiency syndrome. Am J Med 85:428–431, 1988

Robinson JD: Vanadate inhibition of brain (Ca + Mg)-ATPase. Neurochem Res 6:225–232, 1981

Rodriguez CE, Wolfe AL, Bergstrom VW: Hypokalemic myocarditis. Am J Clin Pathol 20:1050–1057, 1950

Roelofsen B: The (non)specificity in the lipid requirement of calcium-and (sodium plus potassium)-transporting adenosine triphosphatases. Life Sci 29: 2235–2247, 1981

Roose SP, Bone S, Haidorfer C, et al: Lithium treatment in older patients. Am J Psychiatry 136:843–844, 1979a

Roose SP, Nurnberger JI, Dunner DL, et al: Cardiac sinus node dysfunction during lithium treatment. Am J Psychiatry 136:804–806, 1979b

Rosenbaum AH, Barry M: Positive therapeutic response to lithium in hypomania secondary to organic brain syndrome. Am J Psychiatry 132:1072–1073, 1975

Ross CA, Meldolesi J, Milner TA, et al: Inositol 1,4,5-triphosphate receptor localized to endoplasmic reticulum in cerebellar Purkinje neurons. Nature 339:468–470, 1989

Ross DR, Coffey CE, Ferren EL, et al: "On-off" syndrome treated with lithium carbonate: a case report. Am J Psychiatry 138:1626–1627, 1981

Rothstein G, Clarkson DR, Larsen W, et al: Effect of lithium on neutrophil mass and production. N Engl J Med 298:178–180, 1978

Ryan WG, Richards JM, Lee JV: Characteristics of the in vivo RBC: plasma lithium ratio in clinical setting. Bull Psychiatry 26:533–537, 1989

Rybakowski J, Strzyzewski W: Red-blood-cell lithium index and long-term maintenance treatment. Lancet 1:1408–1409, 1976

Rybakowski J, Frazer A, Mendels J, et al: Erythrocyte accumulation of the lithium ion in control subjects and patients with primary affective disorder. Commun Psychopharmacol 2:99–104, 1978a

Rybakowsky J, Frazer A, Mendels J: Lithium efflux from erythrocytes incubated in vitro during lithium carbonate administration. Commun Psychopharmacol 2:105–112, 1978b

Rybakowski J, Potok E, Strzyzewski W: Erythrocyte membrane adenosine triphosphatase activities in patients with endogenous depression and healthy subject. Eur J Clin Invest 11:61–64, 1981

Rybakowski JK, Amsterdam JD: Lithium prophylaxis and recurrent labial Herpes infections. Lithium 2:43–47, 1991

Sacchetti E, Bottinelli S, Bellodi L, et al: Eryrocyte plasma lithium ratio (letter). Lancet 1:908, 1977

Saitoh T, Schwartz JH: Phosphorylation-dependent subcellular translocation of a Ca^{2+}/calmodulin-dependent protein kinase produces an autonomous enzyme in aplasia neurons. J Cell Biol 100:835–842, 1985

Saitoh Y, Yamamoto H, Fukuraga K, et al: Inactivation and reactivation of the multifunctional calmodulin-dependent protein kinase from brain by autophosphorylation and dephosphorylation: involvement of protein phosphatases from brain. J Neurochem 49:1286–1292, 1987

Salama AA: Complete heart block associated with mesoridazine and lithium combination. J Clin Psychiatry 48:123, 1987

Saltiel AR, Fox JA, Sherline P, et al: Insulin-stimulated hydrolysis of a novel glycolipid generates modulators of CAMP phosphodiesterase. Science 233:967–972, 1986

Samson JA, Simpson JC, Tsuang MT: Outcome studies of schizoaffective disorders. Schizophr Bull 14:543–554, 1988

Santella RN, Rimmer JM, MacPherson BR: Focal segmental glomerulosclerosis in patients receiving lithium carbonate. Am J Med 84:951–954, 1988

Saran AS: Antidiabetic effects of lithium. J Clin Psychiatry 43:383–384, 1982

Sarantidis D, Waters D: A review and controlled study of cutaneous conditions associated with lithium carbonate. Br J Psychiatry 143:42–50, 1983

Sashidharan SP, McGuire RJ: Recurrence of affective illness after withdrawal of long-term lithium treatment. Acta Psychiatr Scand 68:126–133, 1983

Sautter F, Garver D: Familial differences in lithium responsive versus lithium non-responsive psychoses. J Psychiatr Res 19:1–8, 1985

Sautter FJ, McDermott BE, Garver DL: A family study of lithium-responsive psychosis. J Affect Disord 20:63–69, 1990

Sawada M, Ichinose M, Maeno T: Protein kinase C activators reduce the inositol triphosphate-induced outward current and the Ca^{2+}-activated outward current in identified neurons of aplasia. J Neurosci Res 22:158–166, 1989

Schildkraut J: The catecholamine hypothesis of affective disorder: a review of supporting evidence. Am J Psychiatry 122:509–522, 1965

Schildkraut JJ: Pharmacology—the effects of lithium on biogenic amines, in Lithium: Its Role in Psychiatric Research and Treatment. Edited by Gershon S, Shopsin B. New York, Plenum Press, 1973, pp 51–73

Schildkraut JJ, Orsulak PJ, Schatzberg AF, et al: Toward a biochemical classification of depressive disorders, I: differences in urinary excretion of MHPG and other catecholamine metabolites in clinically defined subtypes of depressions. Arch Gen Psychiatry 35:1427–1433, 1978

Schlagerhauf G, Tupin J, White RB: The use of lithium carbonate in the treatment of manic psychoses. Am J Psychiatry 123:201–207, 1966

Schmalzing G: Coupling of lithium Ca^{2+}/distribution to the plasma membrane potential of rat cortical synaptosomes. J Biol Chem 261:650–656, 1986

Schmitt CA, McDonough AA: Developmental and thyroid hormone regulation of two molecular forms of Na^{+}-K^{+}ATPase in brain. J Biol Chem 261:10439–10444, 1986

Schottstaedt WW, Grace WJ, Wolff HG: Life situations, behavior, attitudes, emotions and renal excretions of fluid and electrolytes, II: retention of water and sodium; diuresis of water. J Psychosom Res 1:147–152, 1956a

Schottstaedt WW, Grace WJ, Wolff HG: Life situations, behavior, attitudes, emotions and renal excretion of fluid and electrolytes, III: diuresis of fluid and electrolytes. J Psychosom Res 1:203–211, 1956b

Schottstaedt WW, Grace WJ, Wolff HG: Life situations, behavior, attitudes, emotions and renal excretion of fluid and electrolytes, IV: situations associated with retention of water, sodium and potassium. J Psychosom Res 1:287–291, 1956c

Schou M: Biology and pharmacology of the lithium ion. Pharmacol Rev 9:17–58, 1957

Schou M: Lithium in psychiatric therapy: stock-taking after ten years. Psychopharmacologia 1:65–78, 1959

Schou M: Electrocardiographic changes during treatment with lithium and with drugs of the imipramine-type. Acta Psychiatr Scand Suppl 39:168–171, 1963a

Schou M: Normothymetics: "Mood normalizers." Br J Psychiatry 109:803–809, 1963b

Schou M: Lithium in psychiatric therapy and prophylaxis. J Psychiatr Res 6:67–95, 1968

Schou M: Prophylactic lithium maintenance treatment in recurrent endogenous affective disorders, in Lithium: Its Role in Psychiatric Research and Treatment. Edited by Gershon S, Shopsin B. New York, Plenum Press, 1973, pp 269–294

Schou M: Lithium in the treatment of other psychiatric and non-psychiatric disorders. Arch Gen Psychiatry 36:856–859, 1979

Schou M: Problems of lithium prophylaxis: Efficacy, serum lithium, selection of patients. Biol Psychiatry 160:30–37, 1981

Schou M, Juel-Nielsen N, Strömgren E, et al: The treatment of manic psychoses by the administration of lithium salts. J Neurol Neurosurg Psychiatry17:250–260, 1954

Schou M, Juel-Nielsen N, Strömgren E, et al: Behandling of maniske psykoser med lithium. Ugeskrift Larger 117:93–101, 1955

Schou M, Amdisen A, Eskajaer-Jensen S, et al: Occurrence of goiter during lithium treatment. Br Med J 3:710–713, 1968

Schramm M, Selinger Z: Message transmission: receptor controlled adenylate cyclase system. Science 225:1350–1356, 1984

Schreiber G, Avissar S, Aulakh CS, et al: Lithium-selective alteration of the function of brain versus cardiac Gs protein. Neuropharmacology 29:1067–1071, 1990

Schreiber G, Avissar S, Danon A, et al: Hyperfunctional G proteins in mononuclear leukocytes of patients with mania. Biol Psychiatry 29:273–280, 1991

Schwartz G, Lopez-Toca R: Continued lithium treatment after myocardial infarction (letter). Am J Psychiatry 139:255, 1982

Scott M, Reading HW: A comparison of platelet membrane and erythrocyte membrane adenosine triphosphatase specific activities in affective disorders. Biochem Soc Trans 6:642–644, 1978

Secunda SK, Swann A, Katz MM, et al: Diagnosis and treatment of mixed mania. Am J Psychiatry 144:96–98, 1987

Segal RL, Rosenblatt S, Eliasoph I: Endocrine exophthalmos during lithium therapy of manic-depressive disease. N Engl J Med 289:136–138, 1973

Sen AK, Post RL: Stoichiometry and localization of adenosine triphosphate-dependent sodium and potassium transport in the erythrocyte. J Biol Chem 239:345–352, 1964

Sengupta N, Datta SC, Sengupta D, et al: Platelet and erythrocyte-membrane adenosine triphosphatase activity in depressive and manic-depressive illness. Psychiatry Res 3:337–344, 1980

Sengupta N, Datta SC, Sengupta D: Platelet and erythrocyte membrane lipid and phospholipid patterns in different types of mental patients. Biochem Med 25:267–275, 1981

Servant D, Danel T, Goudemand M: Lithium therapy in carbamazepine-induced agranulocytosis (letter). Am J Psychiatry 145:381, 1988

Shaikh IM, Lau BWC, Siegfried BA, et al: Isolation of digoxin-like immunoreactive factors from mammalian adrenal cortex. J Biol Chem 266:13672–13678, 1991

Shapira R, Silberberg SD, Ginsburg S, et al: Activation of protein kinase C augments evoked transmitter release. Nature 325:58–60, 1987

Shaw CM, O'Keeffe R, MacSweeney DA, et al: 3-methoxy-4-hydroxyphenylglycol in depression. Psychol Med 3:333–336, 1973

Shaw DM: Mineral metabolism, mania, and melancholia. Br Med J 2:262–267, 1966

Sheard MH, Marini JL, Bridges CI, et al: The effect of lithium on impulsive aggressive behavior in man. Am J Psychiatry 133:1409–1413, 1976

Sherman WR, Leavitt AL, Honchor MP, et al: Evidence that lithium alters phosphoinositide metabolism: chronic administration elevates primarily d-myoinositol-l-phosphate in cerebral cortex of the rat. J Neurochem 36:1947–1951, 1981

Sherman WR, Munsell LY, Gish BG, et al: Effects of systematically administered lithium on phosphoinositide metabolism in rat brain, kidney and testis. J Neurochem 44:798–807, 1985

Sherman WR, Gish BG, Honchar MP, et al: Effects of lithium on phosphoinositide metabolism in vivo. Fed Proc 45:2639–2646, 1986

Shields SM, Ingebritsen TS, Kelly PT: Identification of protein phosphatase l in synaptic junctions: dephosphorylation of endogenous calmodulin-dependent kinase II and synapse-enriched phosphoproteins. J Neurosci 5:3414–3422, 1985

Shopsin B: Effects of lithium on thyroid function. A review. Dis Nerv Syst 31:237–244, 1970

Shopsin B, Friedmann R, Gershon S: Lithium and leukocytosis. Clin Pharmacol Ther 12:923–928, 1971a

Shopsin B, Kim SS, Gershon S: A controlled study of lithium vs. chlorpromazine in acute schizophrenics. Br J Psychiatry 119:435–440, 1971b

Shukla S, Mukherjee S: Lithium simplex chronicus during lithium treatment. Am J Psychiatry 141:909–910, 1984

Shukla S, Mukherjee S, Decina P: Lithium in the treatment of bipolar disorders associated with epilepsy: an open study. J Clin Psychopharmacol 8:201–204, 1988

Siegelbaum SA, Camardo JS, Kandel ER: Serotonin and cyclic AMP close single K^+ channels in aplasia sensory neurons. Nature 299:413–417, 1982

Silverstone T: Response to bromocriptine distinguishes bipolar from unipolar depression. Lancet 1:903–904, 1984

Silvestri A, Santonastaso P, Paggiarin D: Alopecia areata during lithium therapy: a case report. Gen Hosp Psychiatry 10:46–48, 1988

Simmons DA, Winegard AI: Mechanism of glucose-induced (Na$^+$, K$^+$)-ATPase inhibition in aortic wall of rabbits. Diabetologia 32:402–408, 1989

Simon ML, Strathmann MP, Gautan N: Diversity of G proteins in signal transduction. Science 252:802–804, 1991

Simpson GM: Tardive dyskinesia. Br J Psychiatry 122:618, 1973

Singer I, Rotenberg D: Mechanisms of lithium action. N Engl J Med 289:254–260, 1973

Singer K, Chen R, Schou M: A controlled evaluation of lithium in the premenstrual tension syndrome. Br J Psychiatry 124:50–51, 1974

Singh MM: A unifying hypothesis on the biochemical basis of affective disorders. Psychiatr Q 44:706–724, 1970

Sivadon P, Chanoit P: Employment of lithium in psychomotor agitation: presentation of one clinical experience. Ann Médico-Psychologiques 113:790–796, 1955

Sivilotti L, Nistri A: GABA receptor mechanisms in the central nervous system. Prog Neurobiol 36:35–92, 1991

Sjögren A, Florén C-H, Nilsson Å: Magnesium, potassium and zinc deficiency in subjects with type II diabetes mellitus. Acta Med Scand 224:461–465, 1988

Skinner GRB: Lithium ointment for genital Herpes (letter). Lancet 2:288, 1983

Skinner GRB, Harley C, Buchan A, et al: The effect of lithium chloride on the replication of Herpes Simplex virus. Med Microbiol Immunol 168:139–148, 1980

Sletten IW, Gershon S: The premenstrual syndrome: a discussion of its pathophysiology and treatment with lithium ion. Compr Psychiatry 7:197–200, 1966

Small JG, Small IF, Moore DF: Experimental withdrawal of lithium in recovered manic-depressive patients: a report of five cases. Am J Psychiatry 127:1555–1559, 1971a

Small JG, Small IF, Perez HC: EEG, evoked potential, and contingent negative variations with lithium in manic-depressive disease. Biol Psychiatry 3:47–58, 1971b

Small JG, Kellams JJ, Milstein V, et al: A placebo-controlled study of lithium combined with neuroleptics in chronic schizophrenic patients. Am J Psychiatry 132:1315–1317, 1975

Small JG, Klapper MH, Kellams JJ, et al: Electroconvulsive treatment compared with lithium in the management of manic states. Arch Gen Psychiatry 45:727–732, 1988

Smith SJ, Augustine GJ: Calcium ions, active zones and synaptic transmitter release. Trends Neurosci 11:458–464, 1988

Soderling TR: Protein kinases. J Biol Chem 265:1823–1826, 1990

Sonobe M, Yasuda H, Hisanaga T, et al: Amelioration of nerve Na^+-K^+-ATPase activity independently of myoinositol level by PG_{E1} analogue OP-1206, alpha-CD in streptozocin-induced diabetic rats. Diabetes 40:726–730, 1991

Specht SC: Development and regional distribution of two molecular forms of the catalytic subunit of the Na,K-ATPase in rat brain. Biochem Biophys Res Commun 121:208–212, 1984

Spector R: The specificity and sulfhydryl sensitivity of the inositol transport system of the central nervous system. J Neurochem 27:229–236, 1976

Spector R, Lorenzo AV: Myoinositol transport in the central nervous system. Am J Physiol 228:1510–1518, 1975

Spiegel AM, Rudorfer MV, Marx SJ, et al: The effect of short-term lithium administration on suppressibility of parathyroid hormone secretion by calcium in vivo. J Clin Endocrinol Metab 59:354–357, 1984

Stallone F, Shelley E, Mendlewicz J, et al: The use of lithium in affective disorders, III: a double-blind study of prophylaxis in bipolar illness. Am J Psychiatry 130:1006–1010, 1973

Stauderman KA, Harris GD, Lovenberg W: Characterization of inositol 1,4,5-triphosphate stimulated calcium release from rate cellebellar microsomal fractions. Biochem J 255:677–683, 1988

Stein RS, Beaman C, Ali MY, et al: Lithium carbonate attenuation of chemotherapy-induced neutropenia. N Engl J Med 297:430–431, 1977

Stein RS, Flexner JM, Graber SE: Lithium and granulocytopenia during induction therapy of acute myelogenous leukemia. Blood 54:636–641, 1979

Steiner M, Haskett RF, Osmun JN: Treatment of premenstrual tension with lithium carbonate: a pilot study. Acta Psychiatr Scand 61:96–102, 1980

Stern TA, Lydiard RB: Lithium therapy revisited. Psychiatr Med 4:39–68, 1987

Stokes PE, Shamoian CA, Stoll PM, et al: Efficacy of lithium as acute treatment of manic-depressive illness. Lancet 1:1319–1325, 1971

Strober M, Morrell W, Lampert C, et al: Relapse following discontinuation of lithium maintenance therapy in adolescents with bipolar I illness: a naturalistic study. Am J Psychiatry 147:457–461, 1990

Strom-Olsen R, Weil-Malherebe H: Humoral changes in manic-depressive psychosis with particular reference to the excretion of catecholamines in urine. Journal Mental Science 104:696–704, 1958

Sung RJ, Elser B, McAllister RG Jr: Intravenous verapamil for termination of re-entrant supraventricular tachycardias: intracardiac studies correlated with plasma verapamil concentrations. Ann Intern Med 93:682–709, 1980

Supattapone S, Danoff SK, Theibert A, et al: Cyclic AMP-dependent phosphorylation of a brain inositol triphosphate receptor decreases its release of calcium. Proc Natl Acad Sci USA 85:8747–8750, 1988

Suppes T, McElroy SL, Gilbert J, et al: Clozapine in the treatment of dysphoric mania. Biol Psychiatry 32:270–280, 1992

Suwana AB: Remission of vitiligo and lithium salt medication. J Med Assoc Thai 58:337–338, 1975

Swann AC, Kowlow SH, Katz MM, et al: Lithium carbonate treatment of mania: cerebrospinal fluid and urinary monoamine metabolites and treatment outcome. Arch Gen Psychiatry 44:345–354, 1987

Swann AC, Berman N, Frazer A, et al: Lithium distribution in mania: single-dose pharmacokinetics and sympathoadrenal function. Psychiatry Res 32:71–84, 1990

Swartz CM, Wilcox J: Characterization and prediction of lithium blood levels and clearances. Arch Gen Psychiatry 41:1154–1158, 1984

Sweadner KJ: Overview: subunit diversity in the Na,K-ATPase, in The Sodium Pump: Structure, Mechanism and Regulation. Edited by Kaplas JH, DeWeer P. New York, Rockefeller University Press, 1991, pp 63–76

Swedberg K, Winblad B: Heart failure as a complication of lithium treatment. Acta Med Scand 196:279–280, 1974

Swift JM: The prognosis of recurrent insanity of the manic-depressive type. American Journal of Insanity 64:311–326, 1907

Szabo KT: Teratogenicity of lithium in mice (letter). Lancet 2:849, 1969

Szentistvány I, Janka Z, Szilárd J: Clinical significance of sodium-dependent lithium transport in affective psychoses. Psychiatr Clin 13:57–64, 1980

Takeda K, Noguchi S, Sugino A, et al: Functional activity of oligosaccharide-deficient (Na, K) ATPase expressed in xenopus oocytes. FEBS Lett 238:201–204, 1988

Tang CS, Miller BL: Mechanisms of lithium action: cholinergic/adrenergic balance. Rev Contemp Pharmacoth 4:295–296, 1993

Tang W-J, Gilman AG: Type-specific regulation of adenylyl cyclase by G protein βδ subunits. Science 254:1500–1503, 1991

Tangedahl TN, Gau GT: Myocardial irritability associated with lithium carbonate therapy. N Engl J Med 287:867–868, 1972

Taylor CW, Berridge MJ, Cooke AM, et al: Inositol 1,4,5-trisphosphorothioate, a stable analogue of inositol triphosphate which mobilizes intracellular calcium. Biochem J 259:645–650, 1989

Temple R, Berman M, Robbins J, et al: The use of lithium in the treatment of thyrotoxicosis. J Clin Invest 51:2746–2756, 1972

Thakar JH, Lapierre YD, Waters BG: Erythrocyte membrane sodium-potassium and magnesium ATPase in primary affective disorder. Biol Psychiatry 20:734–740, 1985

Thase ME, Kupfer DJ, Frank E, et al: Treatment of imipramine-resistant recurrent depression, II: an open clinical trial of lithium augmentation. J Clin Psychiatry 50:413–417, 1989

Thomsen K, Olesen OV: Precipitating factors and renal mechanisms in lithium intoxication. Gen Pharmacol 9:85–89, 1978

Tilkian AG, Schroeder JS, Kao JJ, et al: Effect of lithium on cardiovascular performance: report on extended ambulatory monitoring and exercise testing before and during lithium therapy. Am J Cardiol 38:701–708, 1976a

Tilkian AG, Schroeder JS, Kao JJ, et al: The cardiovascular effects of lithium in man: a review of the literature. Am J Med 61:665–670, 1976b

Tisman G, Herbert V, Rosenblatt S: Evidence that lithium induces human granulocyte proliferation: elevated serum vitamin B_{12} binding capacity in vivo and granulocyte colony proliferation in vitro. Br J Haematol 24:767–771, 1973

Tobin RJ, Nemickas R, Scanlon JP, et al: EKG of the month. Ill Med J 146:45–46, 1974

Tollefson GD, Senogles S: A cholinergic role in the mechanism of action of lithium in mania. Biol Psychiatry 18:467–479, 1982

Tomlinson DR, Mayer JH: Reversal of deficits in axonal transport and nerve conduction velocity by treatment of streptozotocin diabetic rats with myoinositol. Exp Neurol 89:420–427, 1985

Torre R, Krompotic E: The in vivo and in vitro effects of lithium on human chromosomes and cell replication. Teratology 13:131–138, 1976

Transbol I, Christiansen C, Baastrup PC: Endocrine effects of lithium, I: hypothyroidism, its prevalence in long-term patients. Acta Endocrinol 87:759–767, 1978.

Tricklebank MD, Singh L, Jackson A, et al: Evidence that a preconvulsant action of lithium is mediated by inhibition of myoinositol phosphatase in rat brain. Brain Res 558:145–148, 1991

Troni W, Carta Q, Cantello R, et al: Peripheral nerve function and metabolic control in diabetes mellitus. Ann Neurol 16:178–183, 1984

Tseng HL: Interstitial myocarditis probably related to lithium carbonate intoxication. Arch Pathol 92:444–448, 1971

Tuomisto J, Tukiainen E: Decreased uptake of 5-hydroxytryptamine in blood platelets from depressed patients. Nature 262:596–599, 1976

Tupin JP, Smith DB, Clanon TL, et al: The long-term use of lithium in aggressive prisoners. Compr Psychiatry 14:311–317, 1973

Urayama O, Shutt H, Sweadner KJ: Identification of three isoenzyme proteins of the catalytic subunit of the Na,K-ATPase in rat brain. J Biol Chem 264:8271–8280, 1989

Valcana T, Timiras PS: Effect of hypothyroidism on ionic metabolism and Na-K activated ATP phosphohydrolase activity in the developing rat brain. J Neurochem 16:935–943, 1969

van der Velde CD: Effectiveness of lithium carbonate in the treatment of manic-depressive illness. Am J Psychiatry 127:345–351, 1970

van der Velde CD, Gordon MW: Manic depressive illness, diabetes mellitus, and lithium carbonate. Arch Gen Psychiatry 21:478–485, 1969

van Praag HM, Korf J, Schut D: Cerebral monoamines and depression. Arch Gen Psychiatry 28:827–831, 1973

Vatal M, Aiyar AS: Phosphorylation of brain synaptosomal proteins in lithium-treated rats. Biochem Pharmacol 33:829–831, 1984

Vernadakis A, Woodbury DM: Electrolyte and amino acid changes in rat brain maturation. Am J Physiol 203:748–752, 1962

Versamis J, MacDonald SM: Manic depressive disease in childhood: a case report. Canad Psychiatr Assoc J 17:279–281, 1972

Vincenzi FF, Larsen FL: The plasma membrane calcium pump: regulation by a soluble Ca^{2+} binding protein. Fed Proc 39:2427–2431, 1980

Vink R, McIntosh TK, Demediuk P, et al: Decrease in total and free magnesium concentration following traumatic brain injury in rats. Biochem Biophys Res Commun 149:594–599, 1987

Vink R, McIntosh TK, Demediuk P, et al: Decline in intracellular free Mg^{2+} is associated with irreversible tissue injury after brain trauma. J Biol Chem 263:757–761, 1988

Volpe P, Krasue K-H, Hashimoto S, et al: "Calciosome," a cytoplasmic organelle: the inositol 1,4,5-triphosphate-sensitive Ca^{2+} store of nonmuscle cells? Proc Natl Acad Sci USA 85:1091–1095, 1988

Voors AW: Lithium in drinking water and atherosclerotic heart disease. Am J Epidemiol 92:164–171, 1970

Waddington JL, Youssef HA: Tardive dyskinesia in bipolar affective disorder: aging, cognitive dysfunction, course of illness, and exposure to neuroleptics and lithium. Am J Psychiatry 145:613–616, 1988

Walaas L, Greengard P: Protein phosphorylation and neural function. Pharmacol Rev 43:299–349, 1991

Walker JB: The effect of lithium on hormone-sensitive adenylate cyclase from various regions of the rat brain. Biol Psychiatry 8:245–251, 1974

Walsh DA, Ashby CD, Gonzalez C, et al: Purification and characterization of a protein inhibitor of adenosine 3:5'-monophosphate-dependent protein kinases. J Biol Chem 246:1977–1985, 1971

Wang YC, Pandey GN, Mandels J, et al: Effect of lithium on prostaglandin F_1-stimulated adenylate cyclase activity of human platelets. Biochem Pharmacol 23:845–855, 1974

Warick LH: Lithium poisoning: report of a case with neurologic, cardiac and hepatic sequelae. West J Med 130:259–263, 1979

Watanabe S, Ishino H, Otsuki S: Double-blind comparison of lithium carbonate and imipramine in treatment of depression. Arch Gen Psychiatry 32:659–668, 1975

Water B, Thaker J, Lapierre Y: Erythrocyte lithium transport variables as a marker for manic-depressive disorder. Neuropsychobiology 9:94–98, 1983

Watson SP, Shipman L, Godfrey PP: Lithium potentiates agonist formation of [³H] CDP-diacylglycerol in human platelets. Eur J Pharmacol 188:273–276, 1990

Weinberg WA, Brumback RA: Mania in childhood: case studies and literature review. Am J Dis Child 130:380–385, 1976

Weiner M, Chausow A, Wolpert E, et al: Effect of lithium on the responses to added respiratory resistances. N Engl J Med 308:319–322, 1983

Weinstein MR: Lithium treatment of women during pregnancy and in the post-delivery period, in Handbook of Lithium Therapy. Edited by Johnson FN. Lancaster, England, MPT Press, 1980, pp 421–429

Weiss H: Über eine neue Behandlungsmethode dea Diabetes mellitus und verwandter Stoffwechselstörungen. Wien Klin Wochenschr 37:1142–1143, 1924

Weissman MM, Myers JK, Harding PS: Prevalence and psychiatric heterogeneity of alcoholism in a United States urban community. J Stud Alcohol 41:672–681, 1980

Wellens JH, Cats VM, Duren DR: Symptomatic sinus node abnormalities following lithium carbonate therapy. Am J Med 59:285–287, 1975

Weller RA, Weller EB, Tucker SG, et al: Mania in prepubertal children: has it been underdiagnosed? J Affect Disord 11:151–154, 1986

Whalley LJ, Scott M, Reading HW, et al: Effect of electroconvulsive therapy on erythrocyte adenosine triphosphatase activity in depressive illness. Br J Psychiatry 137:343–345, 1980

Wharton RN, Fieve RR: The use of lithium in the affective psychoses. Am J Psychiatry 123:706–712, 1966

Whitehead PL, Clark LD: Effect of lithium carbonate, placebo, and thioridazine on hyperactive children. Am J Psychiatry 127:824–825, 1970

Whitworth P, Kendall DA: Effects of lithium on inositol phospholipid hydrolysis and inhibition of dopamine D_1 receptor-mediated cyclic AMP formation by carbachol in rat brain slices. J Neurochem 53:536–541, 1989

Whitworth P, Heal DJ, Kendall DA: The effect of acute and chronic lithium treatment on pilocarpine-stimulated phosphoinositide hydrolysis in mouse brain in vivo. Br J Pharmacol 101:39–44, 1990

Wilbanks GD, Bressler B, Peete CH, et al: Toxic effects of lithium carbonate in a mother and newborn infant. JAMA 213:865–867, 1970

Wilk S, Shopsin B, Gershon S, et al: Cerebrospinal fluid levels of MHPG in affective disorders. Nature 235:440–441, 1972

Wilson JR, Kraus ES, Bailas MM, et al: Reversible sinus-node abnormalities due to lithium carbonate therapy. N Engl J Med 294:1223–1224, 1976

Wolff J, Berens SC, Jones AB: Inhibition of thyrotropin-stimulated adenyl cyclase activity of beef thyroid membranes by low concentration of lithium ion. Biochem Biophys Res Commun 39:77–82, 1970

Wolpert EA: Nontoxic hyperlithemia in impending mania. Am J Psychiatry 134:580–582, 1977

Wood AJ, Elphick M, Aronson JK, et al: The effect of lithium on cation transport measured in vivo in patients suffering from bipolar affective illness. Br J Psychiatry 155:504–510, 1989

Worrall EP: Lithium in Huntington's chorea (letter). Lancet 2:1323, 1974

Worrall EP, Moody JP, Peet M, et al: Controlled studies of the acute antidepressant effects of lithium. Br J Psychiatry 135:255–262, 1979

Worthley LI: Lithium: Lithium toxicity and refractory cardiac arrhythmia treated with intravenous magnesium. Anaesthesia & Intensive Care 2:357–360, 1974

Wright TL, Hoffman LH, Davies J: Lithium teratogenicity (letter). Lancet 2:876, 1970

Yassa R, Nair V: Prophylaxis and the lithium ratio in bipolar patients. Prog Neuropsychopharmacol Biol Psychiatry 9:423–428, 1985

Yorek MA, Dunlap JA: Resting membrane potential in 41 A3 mouse neuroblastoma cells. Effect of increased glucose and galactose concentrations. Biochim Biophys Acta 1061:1–8, 1991

Yorek MA, Dunlap JA, Leeney EM: Effect of galactose and glucose levels and sorbinil treatment on myoinositol metabolism Na^+-K^+ pump activity in cultured neuroblastoma cells. Diabetes 38:996–1004, 1989

Yorek MA, Dunlap JA, Stefani MR: Restoration of Na⁺-K⁺ pump activity and resting membrane potential by myoinositol supplementation in neuroblastoma cells chronically exposed to glucose or galactose. Diabetes 40:240–248, 1991a

Yorek MA, Stefani MR, Moore SA: Acute and chronic exposure of mouse cerebral microvessel endothelial cells to increased concentrations of glucose and galactose: effect on myoinositol metabolism, PG_{E2} synthesis, and Na⁺-K⁺-ATPase transport activity. Metabolism 40:347–358, 1991b

Youngerman J, Canino IA: Lithium carbonate use in children and adolescents: a survey of the literature. Arch Gen Psychiatry 35:216–224, 1978

Zakowska-Dabrowska T, Rybakowski J: Lithium-induced EEG changes: relation to lithium levels in serum and red blood cells. Acta Psychiatr Scand 49:457–465, 1973

Zall H, Therman POG, Myers JM: Lithium carbonate: a clinical study. Am J Psychiatry 125:549–555, 1968

Zorumski CF, Bakris GL: Choreoathetosis associated with lithium: case report and literature review. Am J Psychiatry 140:1621–1622, 1983

Zucker RS, Lando L: Mechanism of transmitter release: voltage hypothesis and calcium hypothesis. Science 231:574–579, 1986

Zurgil N, Yarom M, Zisapel N: Concerted enhancement of calcium influx, neurotransmitter release and protein phosphorylation by a phorbol ester in cultured brain neurons. J Neurosci 19:1255–1264, 1986

Zusky PM, Biederman J, Rosenbaum JF, et al: Adjunct low dose lithium carbonate in treatment-resistant depression: a placebo-controlled study. J Clin Psychopharmacol 8:120–124, 1988

Index